Conciliation and Mediation in the NHS

a practical guide

Bob Debell

RADCLIFFE MEDICAL PRESS

©1997 Bob Debell

Radcliffe Medical Press Ltd
18 Marcham Road, Abingdon, Oxon OX14 1AA, UK

Radcliffe Medical Press, Inc.
141 Fifth Avenue, New York, NY 10010, USA

British Library Cataloguing in Publication Data

A catalogue record for this book is available from the British Library.

ISBN 1 85775 231 7

Library of Congress Cataloging-in-Publication Data is available.

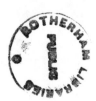

Typeset by Marksbury Multimedia Ltd
Printed and bound by Biddles Ltd, Guildford and King's Lynn

Contents

About the author   v

Introduction   vii

1 Conciliation – mediation – arbitration – what's the difference?   1

2 Summary of the new NHS complaints procedure   5

3 Where can conciliation work?   11

4 What about mediation?   17

5 Preparing the parties to meet   22

6 The conciliation meeting   31

7 The processes of conciliation and mediation   38

8 Listening techniques   42

9 Using body language   51

10 Benefits and shortfalls of conciliation   65

11 When conciliation may not work   74

12 Communicating with the parties to the conciliation process   77

Appendix 1 – Flow chart of the conciliation process   80

Appendix 2 – Check list for the conciliator   82

Glossary   84

Further reading   87

Index   88

(Illustrations by Andrew J S Shaw)

About the author

Bob Debell has spent the whole of his working life in the service industry sector. He was a trainer with the Hotel and Catering Industry Training Board as early as the mid 1960s. He has maintained a keen interest in the development of people's skill, technique and knowledge since that time. He gained training, personnel and general management experience with Hertz Rent A Car international operations and International Computers Ltd. He is multi-lingual and a serious student and exponent of the effective implementation of change across cultural divides. He is the author of the Really Useful Guides to the Single Market and a number of management and business articles. From the late 1970s to the mid 1980s he was variously Human Resource Director and Marketing Operations Director with BL Cars. For a number of years since then he has operated as an independent trainer. From the early 1990s to the present time he has specialized in the provision of training in management and customer care skills to NHS providers. He is now Managing Director of Pragmatic Training Services Ltd.

Introduction

This book is intended to help all those persons throughout the National Health Service (NHS) who become involved in resolving complaints. Some of those people will be specifically nominated to fulfil the formal role of conciliator. Some will be volunteers, giving their time freely to help patients and the NHS to resolve their differences. Some will be front line staff, employees of the NHS who deal with patients on a day-to-day basis and want to improve the quality of care provided to patients. Most of the people involved will, I hope, find that the essence of conciliation is applied common sense.

In researching the subject of conciliation, it was necessary to dig long and hard into the depths of experiences gained in areas other than the NHS. There is very little recorded experience of the use of conciliation within the NHS. Even Relate, which is probably the most experienced operator of conciliation services in the UK, if not the world, was unable to supply any process specification for conciliation. The research involved discussions with the United Nations and ACAS. At the end of the day, it was detailed interviews with experienced conciliators which highlighted the steps to conciliation. Those steps are offered as a guide, but not suggested as a rigid procedure, to help NHS conciliators and employees to achieve the positive results which conciliation is capable of facilitating.

It was very encouraging to find a number of personalities throughout the NHS who had extensive, and successful, experience of conciliation and mediation in resolving differences between complainants and NHS providers. I do believe that the 'introduction' of conciliation to NHS complaints procedures is largely a consolidation of previous good practice. I do also believe that it will benefit all users and employees of the NHS to spread that good practice liberally throughout the service.

Mediation employs very much the same skills as conciliation. The differential which this book introduces, namely that conciliation is largely the province of lay persons, whilst mediation requires a more directive, expert approach is, I think, helpful.

I do suggest that this is not necessarily a book to be read from cover to cover, but rather to be used as a reference base. The structure of the book is intended to provide specific advice on a variety of aspects of conciliation and mediation, chapter by chapter. Researching and preparing the material for the book was a particularly enjoyable experience, which has already proven to be useful in my daily work of training.

Bob Debell
April 1997

1

Conciliation – mediation – arbitration – what's the difference?

Conciliation is a very fashionable technique. The UK legal system has already introduced a requirement for mediation in the Family Law division. The new divorce laws will require every legal practice offering a divorce service to offer mediation to divorcing couples. The objective will be to ensure that the couples agree the division of wealth, family and pets before going to court.

The holiday industry offers an arbitration service to customers who complain. Here the objective is to reach agreement on compensation for holidaymakers whose holiday has gone badly wrong. The service is offered by an industry wide organization which is, in effect, a quasi statutory body.

All over the world arbitration, mediation or conciliation is being introduced to settle disagreements varying from civil war to golf club membership. Now both mediation and conciliation are to be used within the NHS: mediation to resolve situations where a clinical or medical professional and his patient disagree over a treatment and conciliation where any NHS provider and a complainant cannot reach agreement after a complaint against the provider.

So what is this wonderful, new tool for all NHS providers? The dictionary is a good starting point. The unabridged version of Webster's Third New International Dictionary defines the three as follows:

- Arbitration – The hearing and determination of a case between parties in controversy by a person or persons chosen by the parties or appointed under statutory authority instead of by a judicial tribunal appointed by law.
- Mediation – Intervention between conflicting parties or viewpoints to promote reconciliation, settlement, compromise or understanding; intervention of one power between other powers at their suggestion to conciliate differences between them
- Conciliation – The intervention in a dispute by an outsider who seeks to achieve agreement between the disputing parties; the mediation of a (labour) dispute by a third party, governmental or private, having no

power to compel settlement but relying only on persuasion and suggestion.

Thus the dictionary appears to use each of the three to define the other. So how can the NHS practitioner, manager or employee distinguish between the three? For the purposes of this book, which attempts to describe the practical use of mediation and conciliation within an NHS Trust, practice or administrative office, the following definitions will be used:

- Arbitration is the use of an outside body to make a judgement on a dispute between two parties. The judgement will be reached after reasonable discussion between the arbitrator and the parties. The judgement will, in effect, be a decision by the arbitrator. That judgement will be binding on both parties.
- Mediation is the use of reasonable discussion between the parties, led by an outside person. The mediator will have expert knowledge of the matter in dispute. Generally the matter in dispute will be a technical matter. The agreement reached between the parties, under the guidance of the mediator, will be regarded as a final position, and as such is expected to be accepted by both parties. The acceptance will, however, be short of the status of legally binding.
- Conciliation is the use of discussion, persuasion and communication skills, particularly listening, by a lay person who has no knowledge of the matter in dispute or of the parties involved. The conciliator will not adopt any stance or personal view, but will attempt to assist the parties to achieve their own agreement.

Thus the three techniques can be summarized as arbitration being a binding judgement, mediation being an expert-assisted agreement and conciliation a discussion-led compromise.

There are some examples of each available. Arbitration is best known for its role in the settlement of industrial disputes. In the UK, ACAS (Arbitration, Conciliation and Advisory Service) is a Quango and will offer neutral premises on which the employer and employee representatives can meet. Typically the two groups will spend some hours in separate rooms with ACAS officials acting as go-betweens. Often the discussions are given the 'heroic' stature of lasting all night. At the end the agreement is almost always a compromise, often a 'meeting in the middle'. Once agreement is achieved on an acceptable result, the parties sign a document which makes that agreement binding. In some cases the parties have to obtain the acceptance of colleagues or members.

In some countries the 'compromise' element is not allowed. 'Pendulum arbitration' requires that the arbitrator eventually decides to impose an agreement in full favour of one party, and totally against the other. Thus in England, if the employer is offering a 2% pay rise, and the union is demanding 5%, the agreement would normally be at about 3.5%. In Australia, their equivalent of ACAS would agree with either the employer's 2% or the union's 5%. Once the decision was made, both parties would have to accept the result absolutely. The effect tends to be that very few disputes actually go to the Australian equivalent of ACAS.

Mediation is the main technique used by the United Nations in attempting to resolve major disputes between countries, or between different factions within a country. In the former Yugoslavia for example, the mediators were political and military experts such as David Owen and General Michael Rose. These mediators used their military and political expertise to attempt to persuade the various groups to accept compromise distributions of territory.

Relate, formerly known as the Marriage Guidance Council, is the best known, and probably most expert, conciliation service in the UK. For many years marriage guidance counsellors have attempted to help couples in the throes of marital dispute. Their aim has normally been to help the couple to reach an agreement to restore their relationship, and continue with the marriage. This is clearly different to the new requirement of the divorce law for mediation to achieve agreement on the details of the break up of the marriage.

These then are the details of arbitration, mediation and conciliation. The skills and techniques involved in arbitration do not have a place in the requirements of the new complaints procedures or medical mediation, and will not be discussed further in this book. The skills and techniques of conciliation and mediation, however, are the key to the success of the NHS procedures and both will be described in depth. Before starting the discussion, it is wise to look at the people who will be involved.

Mediators will be primarily medical or clinical specialists. The case, for example of a dispute over treatment for glue ear, typically whether or not to fit grommets, would be mediated by an ENT specialist. To be credible a mediator must be able to display expert knowledge of the matter in dispute. Conciliators, on the other hand, must be lay persons. The external conciliator must be acceptable to all parties as a neutral, unbiased, honest broker. He will have some difficulty if he is seen as an employee of the NHS provider, or as a representative of the complainant. The conciliatory approach, however, can be used very successfully by practice, trust or health authority employees.

Both mediators and conciliators need to have the right personality. The basic requirements are the same for both approaches. To succeed, a person needs to be above average in terms of patience, calmness and communication skills. The ability to listen, fully and actively, using all the techniques of eye contact, body language, questioning and reflecting requires a people-orientated approach. Any person who is inclined to be strong willed, imposing their view on others, is very unlikely to succeed as a conciliator and may have difficulty in acting as a mediator. A tendency to adversarial relationships, or a quick temper, will also create difficulties. Whilst conciliators can be trained and developed, the raw material in the form of the personality must be right before starting.

2

Summary of the new NHS complaints procedure

COMPLAINT – AN EXPRESSION OF DISSATISFACTION

In May 1994, a review committee led by Professor Alan Wilson of Leeds University, published their report. The committee had reviewed existing methods of handling complaints in all areas of the National Health Service (NHS). In their report the committee basically recommended that a single procedure for complaints handling should be adopted throughout the NHS in the UK. The prime objective of this procedure is to ensure that complainants are satisfied. The basic operating principle is that complaints should be handled through early discussion and face-to-face communication, not consigned to lengthy exchanges of letters or forms.

The good practice that the committee recommended has been accepted by the vast majority of people as the common sense application of good customer care practice to the unique circumstances which prevail in the NHS. In March 1995 the Government published a response called *'Acting on complaints'*. With minor variations, the Government recommended full implementation of the Wilson Committee proposals from 1 April 1996.

The NHS Executive (NHSE) published interim guidelines later in 1995, and issued final guidelines to all sectors of the NHS during March and April 1996. All providers, from the smallest Family Health Services (FHS) practice to the largest trust and the private sector were required to have detailed complaints handling procedures, train all staff, and deal with complaints to a fairly standard level, from 1 April 1996.

Professor Wilson's suggestion of a single procedure was almost achieved. The NHSE, in their final guidelines, gave different timescales for parts of the procedure as applied to the FHS and secondary sectors. These timescale differentials may lead to some difficulties in administering multiple party complaints. Minor changes were also made to accommodate the alternative NHS structures in the various parts of the UK. Overall the whole of the NHS was given an opportunity to introduce a standard, mainly user-friendly, complaints handling procedure during 'local resolution'. Where a complaint moves into the hands of a convenor, panel or the Ombudsman, however, bureaucratic procedures tend to replace good practice. Thus it is absolutely in the interests of the provider to resolve the complaint as locally, and as quickly, as possible.

One important aspect of good complaint management is not clearly specified in the Wilson report and the documents which followed it. Wilson, by calling his report *'Being Heard'* did try to make the point that communication with patients is the best antidote to dissatisfaction. The Government and the NHSE reverted to the original line of a pure complaints procedure in their guidelines on the subject. Good complaints handling is, in effect, good communication. Pro-active, two-way communication with patients is a key to good patient satisfaction. Listening, to both positive and negative feedback, is good customer care. This aspect of listening to compliments as well as complaints is essential both to conciliation and to good complaints handling. Perfect complaints handling, in effect, is prevention through good service and communication.

The procedure has three levels, or stages. Wilson originally called these stages one, two and three. The NHSE very wisely removed the implication of a progressive staging by naming these stages 'Local resolution', 'Independent review' and 'Ombudsman review'. This reduced the likelihood of complainants feeling that they had to proceed to stage two or three if they were, in fact, satisfied at the first stage.

Local resolution, including conciliation, is the real key to success for the whole system. The intention is that the vast majority of complaints will be properly and fully dealt with at the point of first receipt, probably orally, by the person who first receives the complaint. In order to achieve this, three things have to be set in place by the managers of front line staff.

First, the staff need to be trained. The key skills for good complaints handling are listening skills, the ability to offer an appropriate apology, the ability to recognize a complaint, or a complainant, which needs to be referred to another person, and the ability to take appropriate action to satisfy a complainant. As these are all interpersonal skills, the training needs to be interactive. Training by competent managers at work, or group training in a workshop environment, are the most likely routes to success (Case Study 1).

Case Study 1

One ward in an acute hospital had a much higher level of complaints by patients about their food than any other part of the unit. It was discovered that the ward staff had been instructed to always give any patient who complained a standard form, and encourage them to complete it. This was intended to ensure that the blame for the cold or poor food was always passed to the 'right' people and ensure minimum involvement of ward staff. As part of the introduction of changed complaints procedures, the ward nurse manager was trained in the skills of complaints management, including listening and

Case Study 1: *continued*

offering an apology. She was delegated the responsibility to train her own staff to handle complaints on the spot. After three weeks the number of complaints formally registered was reduced by 97%. The total time taken by ward staff to deal with complaints about food was actually considerably reduced. Most important of all the patients, all long stay patients, clearly stated that they believed the food had improved.

Second, the staff must know the rules. Practice or trust protocols should be available so that all staff know exactly the services and standards they can offer to patients. If the standards are known and complied with, the primary objective of preventing complaints by ensuring that all patients know what to expect, allied to staff providing just that standard of service, should ensure a positive acceptance of service by patients and very few complaints. Setting protocols clearly also enables decisions to be made to vary the standard where appropriate (Case Study 2).

Case Study 2

In a general practice there was a rule which stated clearly that patients were required to give 48 hours' notice for a repeat prescription. Very few patients took any notice, two of the partners disagreed with the rule and always intervened if they heard a patient being asked to give notice. There were constant complaints from patients about repeat prescriptions being late. A new practice manager was appointed and she asked all staff and all partners to try a three-month period during which all patients, excepting identifiable emergencies, would be required to wait 24 hours for their repeat scripts. After only one month the reluctant partners commented on the change to their consultations with patients which suffered far fewer interruptions. At the end of three months over 80% of patients were giving at least 24 hours' notice, the complaints had dwindled to virtually zero on this topic, and all the practice partners and staff felt that stress levels were down.

The third requirement is that the managers must motivate their staff to want to resolve patient problems. In practice this is probably easier than it would be in most commercial organizations. The staff who have the highest level of direct patient contact tend to be the non-medically qualified staff, receptionists in the FHS, nursing assistants on the ward, and hotel services staff, etc. These are, in many cases, people who have chosen to work in the NHS because they are caring, gregarious personalities. In the main, they are pleased to be able to help resolve problems for other people in general, and for patients in particular. Thus the job of motivating staff can be comparatively simple for a good manager.

The local resolution of complaints does rely heavily on the front line staff. Wilson stated that 98% of all complaints should be properly and fully dealt with 'on the spot'. The complaints which cannot be dealt with in this way tend to be either the more serious matters, or those cases where the nature of the complainant is such that they will not be satisfied. The front line staff have to recognize both these situations and pass the complaint quickly to a person who has been designated to handle and manage complaints locally.

In a practice this would logically be the practitioner, partner or practice manager. In an acute trust, one person in each directorate, or even each ward, should be designated to handle such complaints. In an ambulance trust it could well be a superintendent. There could be a temptation to appoint a special person. This would, indeed, be helpful for a large unit. The culture of the unit should, however, be encouraged to think of that person as a positive input to help both staff and patients to improve communication, service quality and satisfaction. It is difficult to achieve this if the designated person is given a negative job title such as 'Complaints Manager'. Positive all-round results will be better served with a job title such as 'Patient Services Manager', 'Quality Manager' or 'Patients' Advocate'. In truth, there is often no reason to create a special job title at all. If the person designated already has a job title such as 'Nursing Director' or 'Practice Manager', why change it?

The person designated to deal with those more complex complaints will need to use a variety of techniques. Conciliation is clearly one and is best used at a very early stage in the handling of the complaint. The temptation to keep conciliation back as a last resort tool will often result in failure. Far more important in most cases is the ability of the manager to adopt a conciliatory approach. Using the style of conciliation from the first moment of contact will ensure positive satisfaction of the complainant in the vast majority of cases. The techniques described above of handling complaints for front line staff are clearly a part of the designated person's battery of skills, simply used at a more expert level.

Investigation of complaints will be a major part of the work involved in complaint management at this level. Good investigation needs to be done quickly if it is to succeed. The Wilson procedure helps this by setting tight deadlines for completion of local resolution. Medical professionals, used to averaging 18 months to resolve a complaint, will suffer a degree of 'culture shock' by having to complete resolution within 22 working days, approximately one month.

Written acknowledgements of complaints must also be sent where it is appropriate to do so. In accordance with the Patients' Charter which preceded the new complaints procedure, each written complaint must receive a written response signed by the chief executive. Good managers of complaints will avoid the temptation to interpret this as suggesting that written complaints are more serious than verbal complaints. Wilson stated quite clearly, and correctly, that all complaints, written or verbal, should receive the same consideration and sensitive treatment. The letter which finalizes local resolution must include details of the right of the complainant to request that an independent review be made of their complaint if they remain dissatisfied. Here, as at all stages of the handling of the complaint, the complainant must be made aware of the help available to them, particularly through the Community Health Council (CHC), to progress their complaint.

If the complainant is dissatisfied after local resolution, the request for an independent review will be passed to a convenor who will decide whether or not to convene a review panel. The convenor will be a non-executive director of the trust, health authority or health board. The convenor has to decide, within one month for a trust complaint, two weeks for an FHS complaint, whether or not to convene a panel. A panel will be convened only if the convenor decides that a panel can add value to the case of the complaint. If it is believed that everything possible and reasonable has already been done at local resolution then no panel will be convened. In the first six months of the new procedure, the vast majority of panel requests were in fact returned by the convenor for the trust or practice to attempt further local resolution. Often these have been on the grounds that not everything, particularly the use of conciliation, has been attempted within the first local resolution.

The convenor, or the panel, should use a conciliatory approach to their work. By adopting such a user-friendly approach, a panel may be able to achieve satisfaction of the complaint to the benefit of all parties. If the panel adopt a tribunal style to their work they are unlikely to achieve any positive outcome. Bureaucracy is not a good way to handle dissatisfied patients.

The panel, if convened, will produce a report, strictly adhering to terms of reference set by the convenor. The panel is a subcommittee of the board of the trust, health authority or health board and can make recommendations for any action it believes will help to satisfy the complainant, whilst being scrupulously fair to the complained against. If the complainant is dissatisfied with either the convenor's decision, or the panel's report, he can appeal to the Health Service Commissioner (the Ombudsman).

The message for any FHS practice or trust is really very simple. Local resolution provides an opportunity to deal with a complaint properly and fully at a local level. Convenors, panels and the Ombudsman are best avoided by the front line staff properly satisfying complainants at the earliest possible moment. A conciliatory approach to complaints, and the use of an experienced conciliator, can pay enormous dividends in saved time and reduction of stress for all concerned.

3

Where can conciliation work?

There are two levels at which conciliation techniques can positively help with the handling of a complaint. The first, and probably the most important, is the use of a conciliatory approach by all the persons involved in dealing with the complaint during local resolution. The second is the introduction of a lay conciliator to act as an honest broker and help the parties involved to reach agreement from an 'outsider' standpoint.

The conciliatory approach consists of using the techniques described throughout this book, almost casually, from the moment of first contact with the complainant right through to the tone of the letter which finalizes local resolution. The use of full active listening techniques (Chapter 8) is probably the key to success. It is very unlikely that there will ever be any complaint situation in which the use of a conciliatory approach is not beneficial. This book will concentrate on the techniques and skills of conciliation, mainly describing them in the context of use by a lay conciliator, and the use of these techniques in a conciliatory approach to all aspects of the handling of complaints. Most importantly, the user-friendly effect of a conciliatory approach by front line staff will maximize positive responses from complainants. This approach will greatly assist the lay conciliator in his further attempts to reach agreement between the parties from an outsider standpoint.

Conciliation, introduced as a major formal part of local resolution, can work in many situations. Generally, an external conciliator will only be brought in to help if it is clear that there is, or may be, difficulty in communicating between the complainant and the complained against. A very important skill for the 'designated person' is to be able to recognize a situation in which such problems may occur. That recognition is best made at a very early stage. Inappropriate attempts to handle the complaint by employees could worsen the situation, and make the conciliator's task more difficult.

A lay conciliator should be introduced where either party is reluctant to enter into face-to-face discussion. In some cases, typically where a patient is complaining about rudeness, for example, the complainant may feel that he does not want to face the rude doctor. Alternatively, a nurse who is 'accused' by a patient of poor professional standards may not wish to face her accuser. In either case, or any situation of hesitancy by either party, the introduction of a lay conciliator is advised. The person who is handling the complaint as a 'designated' person is the most likely to decide to ask a lay conciliator to become involved. The lay conciliator will normally want only the names of the parties, and their contact telephone numbers or addresses. The designated person will almost certainly want to tell the conciliator all the details of the complaint, and the parties involved. The conciliator should not be interested in the tale, but has to find out exactly how the parties themselves feel at this stage. To listen to the practice manager's version of events would be to take the risk of accepting that version as the fact, or truth. The conciliator would then be potentially biased, act as an 'expert' with his own solution, and thus fail to be a genuine 'lay' conciliator (Case Study 3).

Case Study 3

A complaint by a hospital inpatient regarding the attitude of a night nurse is regarded as requiring the help of a conciliator to resolve. The trust medical director compiles a file about the incident, including 10 testimonials from former patients clearly stating that this nurse is the most caring, helpful nurse for miles around. The conciliator is also shown a document indicating that the patient has complained on two previous occasions about staff rudeness. In such a case, it will be difficult for the conciliator to adopt an absolute neutral start point with both the parties: he will be prejudiced from the start to seek a solution in favour of the nurse, not the agreement the two parties may be able to reach. Conciliation success will be compromised from the start.

As a general statement of probability, a conciliator will be able to achieve success where the parties are normal, reasonable human beings, have been reasonably well dealt with in the handling of the case to date, and are prepared to seek a solution. In some cases, where one of the parties feels that they have not been well treated during the handling of a complaint, the mere introduction of a new person can have a beneficial effect. The act of listening should be a major part of handling both parties involved at all stages of the complaint. As the conciliator is bound to listen, the 'maltreated' party may well become conciliatory as a result of the attention received (Case Study 4)

Case Study 4

A patient suffered a mild heart attack at home. A neighbour dialled 999 to call an ambulance. No ambulance responded. A second 999 call

Case Study 4: *continued*

was made 90 minutes later and an ambulance arrived within a few minutes. The patient was taken to the local trust hospital, where he recovered and eventually returned home. The patient's wife complained in writing that no ambulance responded to the first call. The ambulance trust investigated and discovered that an apparent hoax call from an address similar to this case had been made about one and a half hours before the call. It was also discovered that a serious incident had occurred on a nearby motorway at the same time. A series of letters were sent by the trust to the complainant, each adding a little more of the identified facts. The complainant responded to each letter with an upgrade of the complaint. After four exchanges of correspondence, the complainant was accusing the trust of 'nearly killing my husband'. The trust, in its fourth letter, was suggesting that the neighbour was at fault. A lay conciliator from the local health authority was asked to help resolve the impasse. Without any prior knowledge of the problem, he telephoned both the complainant and the local trust superintendent. He explained to both parties that he was an independent, lay person whose role was to listen to the grievances of both parties and try to help resolve the situation to mutual satisfaction. The complainant responded with 'you are the first person to hint at listening to me'. The superintendent's first reaction was 'there may be something in the hoax call, but Mrs B.... will not listen to reason'. The conciliator knew that as both parties had started to move at the initial contact, the conciliation could proceed with a high chance of success.

There are situations which can make conciliation extremely difficult. Any combination of two or more such situations may even render it unwise to attempt conciliation at all. The prime requirement is that both parties must accept the intervention of a third party to conciliate. If either party refuses to talk to the conciliator, then the conciliator cannot proceed. It is impossible to listen unless somebody is trying to communicate.

A second requirement is that all the persons involved in discussion with the conciliator do have the authority to reach and abide by some form of agreement. In most cases it is best if the patient and the complained against are directly involved. Where a different person has to be involved as the complainant's representative, for example in the case of a child, a mentally ill or elderly and confused patient, the conciliator may need to check that the representative does have the full support and confidence of the patient. In the case of the complained against, it may be a practice manager in the primary sector, or a trust representative from secondary care. Here again the conciliator needs to be certain that the person involved is in a position to make decisions which will stick (Case Study 5)

Case Study 5

A patient detained under the Mental Health Act complained that he had been roughly treated, short of assault, by a nurse in a forensic unit. The patient agreed that his brother could act for him in the negotiation of the matter, and signed the relevant waiver of confidentiality. The trust quality director acted as conciliator between the nurse and the brother. After a brief discussion, the brother accepted that the patient had acted irrationally, and the nurse agreed that he had reacted slightly more than was necessary. The parties reached agreement. The brother visited the patient to explain the result. The patient rejected the agreement reached by his brother, and the end result was an escalation of the complaint, and damaged relationships within the patient's family. In this case it would probably have been necessary to gain the patient's written confirmation of acceptance of the result to be negotiated by his brother before starting.

This case also gives a small indication of the special difficulties which can arise for a conciliator where mental illness is involved.

Another situation which can minimize the chances of success will occur if any of the parties involved will not agree to be open and honest with the conciliator. All parties must state that they will be honest. They must agree to tell the conciliator all their beliefs, feelings and emotions. Peculiarly, provided they have agreed to be open and honest, they may then decide to lie, withhold information or deceive the conciliator in any way they wish. It is the initial promise to be open and honest that is important. The conciliator can overcome problems of a lack of candour reasonably easily at later stages.

Yet another difficulty will arise if any party is seriously neurotic, psychotic or addictive. The problem here is comparatively straightforward. The purpose of conciliation is to reach a voluntary agreement, and for the parties to abide by that agreement without any aspect of legal compulsion. Any person affected by such conditions will, of course, very rapidly reach agreement if it suits them at that moment. The problem arises in that they are very likely to renege on that agreement immediately. An agreement reached through conciliation is worthless in such a situation. This again illustrates the special requirements of a complaint involving aspects of mental illness. It is recommended that a conciliator faced with his first case of mental illness should seek professional advice. It is difficult for most people without experience of mental illness to understand and accept some of the finer points of handling communication. The acceptance of mental illness as just one more illness is not a natural reaction, and the conciliator may need to train himself to react in the best and most effective manner.

Alongside this requirement the conciliator must also consider any possibility that one of the parties is prone to physical violence. Such a person may not be suited to the genteel requirements of the conciliation process. The health and safety aspects must also be considered. Not only must the conciliator consider his own safety, but aspects of the law regarding employers' responsibility will also come into play.

Difficulties can also occur if the parties and the conciliator are unable to communicate in a common language. This is a difficulty which is likely to occur quite frequently in a cosmopolitan society. The real difficulty here comes from the lack of properly skilled interpreters. Carrying on any form of communication through an interpreter requires attention to detail by both parties and by the conciliator. The real need is not simply to translate the words, but to interpret the nuances of language and culture. The conciliator will need to study not only the words as spoken by the interpreter, but also the body language of the party for whom the interpreter is acting. In doing this, the conciliator will need to be aware of the differences in body language which occur in other cultures. A simple example is the matter of eye contact. In the Western culture of the NHS, a failure to make any eye contact whilst speaking may well be interpreted as a lack of sincerity. In some Eastern cultures, lowering the eyes away from the other person is a sign of respect. Magistrates, for example, often have to work through interpreters, and frequently come across a situation in which the defendant offers a lengthy and lively response to a question, and the interpreter turns to the magistrate and says simply 'yes'. The true meaning of the reply is lost. This is an extreme example, but the plain fact is that the conciliator must be capable of using a very high standard of communication skills at all stages of the conciliation.

It is useful if the conciliator is able to identify, at an early stage, a clear objective to be achieved through conciliation. This objective does not have to be disclosed to, or agreed with the parties. It is simply a benefit if somebody in the discussions does have a clear idea of where the affair might happily end. The conciliator's view of the end, of course, should be based on his first discussions with the parties, not preconceived.

Conciliation takes time, usually not a great deal of time, an hour or two would be average, but it does take time. If either of the parties, or the conciliator, cannot allow time, preferably on an open-ended basis, then the conciliation will come under uncontrolled pressure to finish and the agreement may not be achieved.

The conciliator must also be accepted by the parties as a neutral, honest, open-minded party to the discussions. If the conciliator is introduced as an employee of the trust, the complainant may, with justification, view him as biased. If he is introduced as a health authority person, the practitioner may believe him to be biased. The conciliator must, therefore, be able to introduce himself to both parties. He should not be put forward by the NHS provider as 'our conciliator'. To achieve this, the conciliator may need to use stationery with the heading 'independent lay conciliator'. In a trust the conciliator will often be an employee of the trust, and should say so as honesty from the conciliator is also important. He should, however, be a skilled communicator and able to convince both parties that he is from a different, uninvolved part of the trust and is capable being neutral, which involves the use of high level communication skills yet again.

Within the NHS arena, it is also essential to ensure that the conciliator offers and maintains a high level of confidentiality to the parties. The conciliator must retain any information given or used during the conciliation process entirely to himself, and assure the parties that their communications are entirely private. The only situation in which the content of the discussion may need to be disclosed to others will occur where, after conciliation has been attempted, legal proceedings are started. Solicitors may make a discovery of documents, at which point any documentary recording of conciliation may have to be handed over. A simple preventative measure would be to mutually destroy any notes, with the parties, at the conclusion of conciliation, thus eliminating any possibility of loss of confidentiality. The precise legal standing of conciliation confidentiality is not as clear as the confidentiality of Family Law mediation. The confidentiality requirement does not apply in the same way to medical mediation: here the normal rules of medical patient confidentiality apply.

In conclusion, then, conciliation can work if the parties are reasonable people, if they all agree to conciliation, and if the conciliator is a skilled communicator. This gives a clear confirmation of the need for the conciliator to start with the right personality, and to develop a high level of communication skill and technique.

4

What about mediation?

Conciliation is non-directive and mediation, on the other hand, is specifically directive. The conciliator starts with the views of the parties, and helps them to reach an agreement that is mutually acceptable. That acceptability is, basically, irrespective of common sense. For example, if one party is prepared to move 99% of the way, and the other party reluctantly moves 1%, even if this end result is clearly unreasonable to a casual observer, if the two parties both accept this irrational result, it does not matter. Conciliation requires only that the parties reach and abide by an agreement – any agreement.

This is not the case for mediation. In mediation, the mediator will have a level of expertise relevant to the matter under dispute. The mediator will use the same skills as the conciliator, but with a degree of guidance towards a result that the mediator himself deems to be reasonable in all the circumstances. Mediation, in the main, will be a technique used to resolve differences of opinion between a medical professional and a patient, or patient's representative, regarding the treatment of the patient. In the mediation arena some new factors come into play: differences of opinion between medical or clinical professionals may play a part; changes to established procedures of treatment may need to be clarified; and new procedures or drugs may also play a part. Media publicity given to new or experimental techniques may cause a patient to demand a procedure which is not yet authorized. Politics may enter the arena, particularly with regard to purchasing decisions by health authorities. All or any of these may lead to a situation in which a mediator may be needed to resolve differences.

So where can mediation work? Mediation has a slightly lower requirement for a reasonable stand by the parties. To some extent, because the mediator will be directive, mediation can deal with more entrenched positions than conciliation. The mediator can be presented as an NHS employee, and still succeed. The mediator can declare his specialist knowledge at the start, indeed the whole purpose of his presence is to use that knowledge and experience. Even so, the mediator must present himself as independent of the case before him. A partner of the GP who has 'refused' treatment would probably not be accepted by the patient. A colleague of the consultant, from the same team which offered a treatment which the patient refuses, is clearly not acceptable. On the other side of the coin, a clinical professional who has published a paper opposing the treatment offered by a doctor would be unacceptable to the doctor. From this it is clear that the person who is to act as mediator should be a respected professional with clear knowledge of the ailment and/or the treatments available. The mediator should, however, be sufficiently removed from the personalities and direct NHS providers in the case to be accepted as neutral.

The points which make it difficult for a conciliator can still cause problems for a mediator. It is essential that both parties agree to the intervention of the mediator. In fact, both parties must accept the expertise of the mediator before he commences work. This may place a special task on the mediator of explaining his expertise and persuading the parties to accept him. The techniques required to achieve this, particularly if the parties resist, is closely akin to the techniques of selling in the commercial world. The first task is to gain acceptance as a person. Listening techniques are the main tool to achieve this. Once accepted as a person, then the professional expertise has to be 'sold'. To convince the clinical or medical professional in the dispute, a short explanation of experience will normally suffice. In some cases the mediator's reputation will go before him.

The patient may not be so easy to convince. Professional qualifications and experience will be a good starting point. It is essential, however, that the patient accepts the mediator as a person with experience, understanding and acceptance of all the factors involved in the case. To do this, the mediator will probably need to give examples of situations in which he has used both, or all, the techniques. In so doing it will be helpful if he can get across the message that different circumstances call for different approaches. A friendly, quiet 'chat' with the patient, or patient representative in the case of a child or other person who is not capable of making their own decisions, should be enough to convince them that the mediator is a person worthy of discussing their problem (Case Study 6).

Case Study 6

A young child was suffering from glue ear. The child had an older sister who had suffered five years earlier, and had benefited from the fitting of grommets. The child's mother was quite clear on the matter: if grommets worked for the first child, they were bound to work for the second. Not so the local ENT specialist. He was of the opinion that the child required no treatment, and should be left to allow spontaneous resolution. Deadlock soon occurred. The GP concerned offered the services of a specialist from another trust, a well known teaching hospital, to mediate. The ENT specialist knew of the reputation of the person concerned and readily accepted that he could act as mediator, and even suggested that he would accept the decision of the mediator

Case Study 6: *continued*

as final. The mother, however, had heard of another child at her local school who had been refused grommets by the same teaching trust and declined to accept his involvement. The proposed mediator contacted the mother and asked her to visit him at his rooms to discuss the matter. The mother agreed, and the mediator started by showing her an article which he had published. The article was entitled 'Grommets – The argument for and against'. On seeing the title the mother accepted the mediator as neutral and he was able to proceed. This case illustrates that a mediator (or a conciliator) may be able to gain acceptance of himself, or of his proposed process, by applying a little persistence even after initial rejection.

The need for a statement by the parties that they will be fully open and honest is not so strong in mediation. A promise to disclose sources of information and bases of decisions will suffice. The need for both parties to have the authority to reach and implement an agreement is, however, paramount. In particular, if the medical professional is not authorized to implement the decision, the mediation cannot succeed. This will be particularly important in the case of a purchasing decision. It is all very well for the surgeon to agree that cosmetic surgery is indicated, but if nobody is prepared to pay for it, then the mediation agreement cannot be implemented. In such cases the persons involved in mediation may need to include the purchaser of services as well as the professionals.

The conciliator must be seen as 'neutral, honest and trustworthy' by both parties. The mediator, on the other hand, must be seen as competent, open and dependable by the parties. He may also need to be seen as authoritative. This can place a requirement for the mediator to look the part. If it is expected by a reasonable group of persons that a specialist should be formally dressed, the mediator will find it difficult to succeed if he wears casual clothing. The argument that casual clothing will make the patient feel at ease is unlikely to prevail.

With a specialist as the mediator, he should be able to cope with, and either overcome or work around any problems such as neurotic, psychotic or addictive patients. The professional authority of the mediator, and the nature of the treatment under discussion, should ensure that the agreement can be implemented even if the patient does change his mind. As the mental health sector is likely to have a higher incidence of cases going to mediation than most, this is an important difference.

The mediator, the parties and any third parties must, of course, be able to devote the necessary time to mediation discussion. In most cases the time needed will be comparatively short. The issues will usually be more clear cut than in conciliation, and will often boil down to a single, easily identified matter of disagreement over one point.

Even the language barrier is easier to overcome in the case of mediation. Much of the discussion will concern technical matters for which there is often a common or similar word. The nuances of language and culture may still exist, but should be clearly identified in advance. Different attitudes towards medical treatments are mostly well known, and provided the cultural background of the parties is identified in advance, the mediator can prepare for such differences (Case Study 7).

Case Study 7

A child patient was diagnosed as suffering from an ailment requiring treatment which might include blood transfusion. The parents, on religious grounds, stated that a blood transfusion was not to be done. The hospital managers decided that if the parents continued to refuse blood transfusion they would ask the local authority welfare section to seek ward of court status. A member of the trust staff, with similar religious beliefs to the parents, was asked to act as mediator. The mediator was made aware of the inevitability of court action, and was given access to legal advice on the likely outcome of that legal action before mediation started. He was, therefore, placed in a situation in which he was given a clear objective to achieve, with little room for manoeuvre. The mediator accepted the task, and was accepted as a mediator by the parents. He gained the parents' partial agreement to the treatment, with a proviso that the transfusion would be used only if deemed essential by a minimum of two experienced surgeons. The trust agreed to the condition and confirmed this in writing. The treatment went ahead successfully. The parents accepted, but made clear their strong dislike of the need for transfusion. The only reason the mediator gained their agreement was the pressure brought to bear regarding the inevitability of the legal action. In another similar case, the parents took their child overseas to avoid the treatment before mediation was invoked. Whilst this case does illustrate again that persistence may lead to a positive benefit, it must be stated that any form of religious belief is often classified at the extreme end of attitude. As such it cannot normally be overturned. This case could be said to have succeeded more because of the pressure from threatened legal action than the particular skill of the mediator.

Thus it is clear that there are distinct differences between mediation and conciliation. Mediation is likely to succeed in situations where there is rejection of medical or clinical treatment, diagnosis or advice by patients. Mediation must not, however, be used as a tool to 'bully' all patients into agreeing with every word a medical professional says. The normal test, namely that a responsible body of professionals would be expected to support the views expressed, needs to be applied before mediation can be implemented with a fair chance of success. Mediation is unlikely to help impose a minority, or experimental, view on patients. The test of overall reasonableness of the outcome is more important than in conciliation. For the balance of this book, the emphasis will be on conciliation, with differences for mediation highlighted where relevant.

5

Preparing the parties to meet

Now that we have identified what conciliation (and mediation) is, and where it may work, the time has come to examine the process which is called conciliation. First it should be clear that conciliation is not a practice that can be easily formed into a standard procedure. Conciliation cannot be made to follow any precise book of rules.

The following process might be described as a 'model' format. In almost every real conciliation, all the steps described here will occur. Sometimes those steps will be in the order illustrated here, sometimes each step will be identifiable as a precise step and sometimes the steps will be intermingled, virtually instantaneous, and pass totally unnoticed. That is the very essence of conciliation. No two attempts to conciliate will ever be the same. We are dealing with human beings, and they are all different.

The process starts, like most human activities, with a period of preparation. Conciliation is really like an iceberg – 90% of the process is not seen. The conciliator will not bring the parties together for discussion until he is confident that there will be conciliatory 'movement' by all parties. To make the process reasonably simple, we have prepared this illustration based on two parties, the complainant and the complained against. In many situations there will actually be more than two parties, which makes the process more complex but does not change the basic principles.

The first contact for the conciliator may be a request to conciliate from the complained against, normally a practice or trust. Sometimes the request may come from the complainant. This will be rare, but is possible. Another possibility is that the request will come from a third party who has become involved in the dispute at an earlier stage, at the request of one of the parties. This could be a health authority, health board or the Community Health Council. The most difficult cases to resolve will probably be those which are generated as a result of the Independent Review Panel Convenor sending a complaint back for further local resolution. These will be cases where the attempts to resolve the dispute have already failed at least once.

The person requesting the conciliator's help is almost certain to want to tell the conciliator what has happened so far. The conciliator will need to resist the temptation to hear the juicy details. If the conciliator is to be a genuinely 'lay' conciliator, he must be totally untarnished with the views of those already involved in trying to resolve the dispute. The conciliator's opening file should be a clean sheet of paper. He must try to start each contact with a 'blank mind'. The mediator, on the other hand, may well prepare a full file of facts including medical notes. He approaches as an expert, not as a 'lay' person.

The conciliator's first two actions should be to contact both the parties, and get their stories from them. The conciliator must be able to listen to those stories in a totally unbiased, neutral, honest broker way. This first contact with each of the two parties is crucial. These communications with the parties will, of course, be conducted quite separately. The conciliator, in the first few moments of each of these contacts, must achieve several aims. First, he must gain acceptance by the parties of his involvement. In some cases this will already have been established by the trust, practice or Heath Authority/Board, but in some cases, the conciliator will need to explain who he is and what his role is. If either of the parties is security conscious, he may have to prove his very identity.

Once he is accepted as a person, the conciliator must prove that he is impartial. Sometimes a simple statement that he is a lay conciliator will be enough. Some parties may instantly regard the conciliator as biased, and will need to be reassured. Comments such as 'I have been asked by the West Heartshire NHS Trust to contact you...' or 'I am the lay conciliator for the Coshington Health Authority' must be avoided. These simple words may instantly cause either party to decide that the conciliator is biased and is there to help the other side. It is much better to use phrases such as 'I am a lay conciliator, available to try to help both yourself and the ...' or 'My role is to listen and help, I do not reach any personal conclusions!'.

The first part of the conciliation process is to listen separately to the two parties' versions of events. To listen fully, without reaching any conclusions, and without bias. To listen openly and thoroughly. The stories that the parties tell the conciliator will be the way the parties see it at the moment of telling. Their stories may vary a great deal from the original complaint or response. In some cases the parties will be much more concerned to recount what has happened since the original incident which was the base cause of the complaint. It has to be recognized that poor or insensitive handling of the complaint by either party is just as likely to be the cause of current disagreement as the original issue.

In some cases, the manager of complaints at the trust, practice or health authority may feel that the complainant has changed, exaggerated or amplified the story since its first telling as a complaint. It is, in fact, quite normal for complainants to change their story of events. The processes of thinking, worrying and becoming frustrated at a lack of response can all contribute to the growth of the complaint in the mind of either party. The conciliator cannot resolve whatever the position was several days, or weeks, ago. The conciliator must work with the current situation.

The best way to listen is to sit in a comfortable place, preferably in a 'lounge' setting. Talking over a desk is really too formal for conciliation, and is better avoided. If it is possible to create the atmosphere of a friendly chat, rather than any formal implication of an interview, the results will be better. Always make sure that the conciliator has the tools to make notes of the conversation. All the listening skills such as body language, eye contact, reflection, questioning etc. should be used to the full. These skills are described in Chapters 7 and 8. The best opening gambit is to use a phrase such as 'Please just tell me everything that has happened, in your own words'. Sometimes the conciliator will have to apologise for asking for a repeat of the story. If the conciliator comes to the case at a late stage, the parties may already have been 'interrogated' by several investigators. Another key point comes in here. The conciliator is *not* seeking to investigate the complaint, he is seeking to get enough of the two stories to enable him to open discussion on the points of agreement, and the points of difference. The investigator will seek to identify the facts of the case, reach a conclusion, and offer an action or 'deal' to conclude the matter. The conciliator must not reach conclusions, and his action is predetermined. His action is to help the two parties to discuss their differences and reach their own agreement. In effect, he is a communication facilitator.

Once the process of a party telling the story is started, it has to be carried through to the end. The conciliator needs all the opinions, views, emotions, facts etc. that the parties hold. The conciliator should make notes, ensuring that all the points made are recorded. When the party has finished, he must ask for more – pregnant pauses can then be used to get even more. When the conciliator is sure that there is no more to come, he should summarize all of it back to the party to get agreement (the listening technique of 'reflection'). The conciliator must not only ensure that he listens to the full story, he must also make sure that the party accepts that his notes are a true summary of the party's story as the party understands it. A useful technique is to repeat the party's points and 'tell the story' just as that. He should make it sound like a story, with a clear beginning, middle and current status (end).

On completing the chat with the first party, the conciliator leaves and then carries out the same process with the other party. These discussions may take place in different rooms within the same building, immediately prior to the conciliator bringing the parties together. The discussions may equally happen in different places and on different days. Sometimes it may be necessary to return to one or both parties to clarify opinions on points raised only by the other party before starting analysis. It is possible, although more difficult, to conduct these conversations on the telephone or even to get the stories in writing. Conciliation works best face to face, but is just about possible to achieve remotely (Case Study 8).

Case Study 8

A lay conciliator was asked by a dentist to intervene in a case of dispute with a patient. The dentist had been trying for some time to resolve the complaint. In his first telephone call to the conciliator, he was clearly agitated, and somewhat angry with the patient's 'unreasonable' approach. He launched into a detailed explanation of the full course of the dental treatment plan. In his view there had been an unreasonable refusal by the Dental Practice Board to authorize part of the proposed course of treatment. He stated several times that he had apologised for the treatment shortfall, and that he had told the patient that it was not his fault. He had given a lengthy tirade on NHS resource shortfalls, a bucketful of instant facts, opinions and attitudes. He appeared to have been very upset by the patient's reaction. The conciliator immediately expected to receive a strong reaction from the patient. The dentist's story was so strong that there really had to be a very emotive patient on the other side. The conciliator prepared himself to talk with the patient, and dialled the number. The patient was very calm, and stated that, in fact, all he wanted was a breakdown of the treatment he could and could not have on the NHS, and a cost for the disallowed treatment. He said that he was very supportive of the dentist, but had difficulty 'getting a word in edgeways'. The conciliator was able to resolve the whole matter with one more telephone call to the dentist. If the conciliator had allowed himself to be influenced by the introductory discussion with the dentist, he might well have adopted a line similar to the dentist's and, as a result, failed to hear what the patient was really saying. Bias was avoided.

When the conciliator has noted both 'stories', the time for analysis has arrived. The conciliator should now take his two lists or stories into a private place and compare them. He will look first of all for areas of agreement. Even in the most difficult situations, there will be at least some points of agreement. For example the parties will at least both say that they met. The time and place may be in dispute, but they both say they met. In most cases there will be a large number of points of agreement. Some may be small, almost insignificant, and some may cover a large portion of the total issue, or handling of the issue, which was the original subject of the complaint.

The conciliator will need to have expert note making skills to capture all the aspects of the issue. The ability to use those notes to analyse the disputed issues into a logical, objective, emotion-free basis for discussion in later meetings is one of the key skills of conciliation. Whichever party is interviewed first, the conciliator is starting with a completely blank sheet. There are no guidelines as to which of the points the party makes can be ignored, and which may become key parts of the conciliation process later. Thus the note taking skill must be to record every detail of both parties' views at the first meetings. Very useful in the conciliation process will be points which one party emphasizes as important issues but the other party fails to mention at all. These may provide the conciliator with items to gain fast 'movement' from the party who had forgotten the item. If he has forgotten it, he may consider it so unimportant that he can concede the point fairly quickly.

It is probably easiest to compile a table, listing items raised in the first column, one party's view in each of the next columns, and a summary of the differences, or agreements, in the fourth column. Once a list of points of agreement and points of difference has been compiled, the size of the problem will become clear. In fact, in most cases, there will be only a small number of clear points of difference. The differences may be very great, but usually few in number.

The next stage is to categorize each point of difference. The categories are (definitions from Merriam Webster Dictionary):

- facts
- opinions
- attitudes.

Facts are:

> An assertion, statement or information containing or purporting to contain something having objective reality.
> The reality of events or things the actual occurrence of which is to be determined by evidence.

Opinions are:

> Belief stronger than impression and less strong than positive knowledge.
> A view or belief that is not demonstrable as fact.
> A belief or view based on interpretation of observed facts and experience.

Attitudes are:

> Preconceived judgement or opinion.
> An opinion or leaning adverse to anything without just grounds or before sufficient knowledge.
> An unreasonable predilection, inclination or objection.

The importance of these definitions for the conciliator is that a *fact* can be objectively proven. An *opinion* may be changed by the use of factual evidence or reasonable discussion. An *attitude* is not capable of change, and the conciliator will have to persuade the other party to ignore it, acknowledge it or simply by-pass it. Thus, the conciliator can use facts as the foundation on which to start the parties 'moving' towards each other. Any disputed fact must cause 'movement' once proven. The opinions are capable of change, and become the real essence of the conciliation. If the parties can be persuaded to 'move' towards each other's point of view on opinions, real progress is made. The attitudes identify the points on which the conciliator cannot expect any movement. These he will not attempt to 'move' towards agreement, but rather plan to use as points to be left in 'agreed disagreement'.

The conciliator's preparation at this stage is to break the dispute down from its emotive whole, to a series of logical, objective parts. The parts can then be dealt with less emotionally. An example of part of a working list of a conciliator's breakdown of his discussions with the parties in a dispute over diagnosis on a home visit by a GP is shown in the Table below:

Item	Dr Brown's view	Mr Smith's view	Analysis
Location of discussion	Mrs Smith's bedroom	Mrs Smith's bedroom	Fact. Agreed. Both clear
Time of discussion	11.30 a.m.	1.00 p.m.	Fact. Disagree Both quite clear
Diagnosis	Mild flu	Pneumonia	Opinion. Disagree Dr very clear, Mrs Smith questioning and unsure
Dr's mood	No comment	Abrupt, rude, very clear	Opinion. Potential disagree
Patient's mood	Neurotic, aggressive, hypochondriac, very strongly put	States worried, ill, (perfectly rational on day of meeting)	Dr – Attitude Mrs Smith – opinion Disagree. **Problem
Treatment	Rest, warmth, light diet	Rest, light food	Opinion. Agreed

In the above example, the conciliator has some points of agreement on which to build. The parties both agree the place of the consultation, and the treatment which was recommended. The disputed fact is about the time of day. This will be a useful point on which to start the parties moving towards each other only if some objective proof of the time can be found. If, for example, an itemized telephone bill showing a call made to or from the house has a time of 12.25 p.m. clearly shown, then both parties can be made to move.

Facts can be difficult to identify. The parties will often introduce an opinion with the words 'It is a fact that ...'. The conciliator should analyse out facts carefully. The only facts that can actually be used to start the process of 'movement' by the parties will be facts which are not only disputed, but for which the conciliator is able to identify and produce clear proof of the true fact. If such proof cannot be found, or will be very difficult to verify, the conciliator will probably do better to classify it as an opinion in the conciliation process. This is more likely to occur where the whole conciliation process has been pre-arranged, and the luxury of time to 'investigate' is not available.

The conciliator's next step is to again meet with the parties separately. The conciliator will open this second part of the discussion by going through each party's story with the other party, highlighting the points on which there is agreement. The tactic here is to achieve agreement from each party that the other party must be right in some aspects. This should be easy to achieve, since the party in discussion has already given the same story on that item. The objective of this part of the discussion is to persuade the parties that they actually have considerable areas of agreement. This can be achieved by simply taking more time over the agreed points than those which are not agreed. It may also be helpful if there is a longer list of agreed points than disputed points – a further justification for really detailed preparation. The analysis is, of course, private to the conciliator. The parties should have an impression of a 'seamless' discussion, and should not in any way realize that the conciliator is using a logical, objective process.

Once the party has accepted that there is some agreement, the time has come to introduce disputed facts. The whole point of the analysis, and the separation of facts from opinions, is to give the conciliator a number of points on which he can achieve movement by both parties before bringing them together for the joint conciliation discussion meeting. If the conciliator has been able to find the objective proof before this second meeting, the process of starting movement should be instant and easy. If the objective proof is not available, then lengthy discussion may ensue. The party must be encouraged to talk, and the conciliator will use a listening technique. In particular, he will use open questions and pregnant pauses followed by specific questions to achieve the desired movement. The key skill is to limit discussion to facts until the party has moved on a fact. It should be possible to move a disputed fact to a point of agreement without the parties having to come together. One useful technique here is to 'hold back' some agreed facts to give a fast 'escape' to new topics once movement has been achieved. This will help the party to accept his own change of view, without loss of face. It is very important not to damage the ego of either party at any stage of conciliation. If the factual proof should be difficult, several 'shuttles' between the parties may be needed. The aim at this stage is to start movement, and keep it going, so that it becomes a comfortable habit for the two, still separate, parties. This momentum can then be maintained by the conciliator as the parties meet, thus helping to ease the parties into movement towards each other's point of view.

Movement by both parties to reach agreement with the conciliator on a disputed fact or facts is essential. The conciliator must keep items on which the parties have opinions and attitudes out of the discussion at this stage. At no time should the conciliator actually use the words 'opinion', 'emotion' or 'attitude' to describe an item. The very use of these words could cause an emotive reaction which might prevent effective conciliation.

Once the parties have both, still separately, moved on a fact, the conciliator can introduce one or more disputed opinions to the discussion. The conciliator may need to describe exactly how or why the other party has a difference on this opinion and will need to introduce other ways of looking at the item. He will use finely honed listening skills, particularly open and specific questions, to keep the party talking until the party gives a clear indication of movement towards the other party's view. If the party has been helped to 'move' on a number of disputed facts, this part of the process may prove quite straightforward. The conciliator needs to use his powers of persuasion, discussion and influence. It is important here to retain the parties' belief that the conciliator is neutral, honest and a lay person. The conciliator must, therefore, not express any personal opinions on the party opinions. Summarizing the party's own opinions, and introducing the other party's opinion on the same item, perhaps in a modified form, is the best technique to use. It may be useful to 'water down' the opposing opinion to achieve movement in stages.

The conciliator must be very attentive at this stage. In a sales interview, salesmen are trained to spot buying signals. This is exactly the skill to be exercised here. In conciliation, the 'buying signal' might be considered as a fish taking a bait. Once the bait is taken, the conciliator winds in the catch, slowly and carefully. In the separate meetings, the conciliator may actually have two 'fishing rods' in use simultaneously.

One 'bait' the conciliator needs to identify is the ideal solution that each party is likely to seek. This is usually fairly easy to establish. Often the party will, in fact, state this as an opening gambit. Once the ideal conclusion is known the conciliator must seek to identify the minimum result each party is likely to accept – this may well be a little more difficult. The conciliator may need to introduce a series of 'what if ...' scenarios to the party and judge reaction. Clear acceptance at this stage is not essential: a lack of outright rejection should be a clear enough indication of eventual acceptability. This identification of minimum and ideal results is essential so that the conciliator can judge the total amount of movement needed by the parties before a conclusion is reached. The differences between their absolute ideals will be the starting point. The difference between their estimated minimum results gives some indication of the likelihood of a successful conclusion.

Identifying the levels of likely acceptable results, and known absolutely unacceptable outcomes, may allow the conciliator to prepare a plan to achieve full conciliation in a series of stages. Whilst the joint conciliation meeting is unlikely to follow a precise plan, if the conciliator is able to prepare a series of 'mini agreements', the final meeting should progress more effectively.

Typical signs of movement might be verbal. Changing from 'I know...' to 'I think...' is a clear signal. A change from 'She did not ...' to 'What did she say she...?' is another example. Signs may be in body language. Unfolding the arms, for example, may be a clear example of acceptance of change. Shrugging the shoulders may also be a good sign, but only if accompanied by positive signs with other body or verbal language. Any movement from a negative to a positive stance is significant.

As soon as there is a small movement, the conciliator will move the discussion to another disputed opinion and attempt again to get some movement. Those items that the conciliator has categorized as attitudes must be carefully kept out of the discussion. Once movement on one or more items has been made, the party can be left in a positive frame of mind ready for the conciliation meeting. The same technique, of course, will be used with both parties.

In mediation, the mediator may also introduce his own opinions or interpretations to the parties at this stage. His own views may be presented as a third party input. A format such as 'Most gynaecologists would recommend....' is a good approach with the patient. This can be modified to 'As you know many of your colleagues in gynaecology would .....' when speaking with the professional.

Once this degree of mutual established movement has been achieved, the conciliator is ready to expose the tip of his iceberg. It is time to bring the parties together in the same room, to discuss their dispute and move towards conciliation.

6

The conciliation meeting

Once the preparation of the parties is complete, they can be brought together to discuss their dispute and reach agreement under the 'chairmanship' of the conciliator. Before they actually come together, some attention must be paid to the setting in which they meet. The easiest way to describe the meeting scene is to discuss the situation which arises when the parties come together in one room, after holding their separate meetings with the conciliator in two other rooms in the same building. It is also easy to assume that perfection can prevail, and that the building in question will have all the facilities required. In reality, many health authorities and trusts will lack the ideal situation, and a compromise as close to this standard as possible will need to be used.

In an extreme case, it is necessary to ensure that both parties perceive themselves as receiving equal treatment from the conciliator. In major arbitration cases, such as civil war or major industrial disputes, the arbitrator has to use a three-room scenario with simultaneous door opening and party entry arranged. Conciliation and mediation rarely require such extreme lengths. It is, however, a good idea to ensure that both parties receive identifiably equal treatment. If the patient is given coffee and biscuits, and the doctor is told to go to the canteen, the doctor is likely to feel that the conciliator is biased.

All the rooms used in conciliation should be as informal, comfortable and user friendly as possible. The joint meeting room is best if it can be made identifiably more informal and friendly than the individual rooms. A move into a slightly warmer room with comfy chairs and an aroma from a coffee machine will help to soothe battered egos. It is also helpful if the walk from the individual rooms to the joint room is quite short. A 'suite' of meeting rooms with 'syndicate' rooms to the sides is probably ideal.

In conciliation, none of the rooms should be set up with conference-style tables; most importantly, the two parties must not be set up to face each other in the confrontational style of a tribunal. Casual seating, coffee tables and circular layout are preferred. Mediation, on the other hand, may well require a more formal setting. Even here, however, a directly confrontational setting is to be avoided. The use of an oval table, or setting the two side tables at an angle of about 140° is better than directly facing.

The conciliator may need to ensure that neither party gains 'territorial advantage' by arriving in the room and sitting down before the other party arrives. In most situations the parties will not be able to enter the room simultaneously from different doors, but ensuring that the first party to enter the room is kept standing until the second party has come in is helpful. The conciliator will need to fully observe body language during the entry to the joint room. The level of aggression or otherwise will be clearly identifiable before the discussion begins. Serving coffee and then taking seats is a useful way to get the parties seated ready for discussion.

Once the parties are seated, the conciliator should open proceedings very briefly. From this point forward, he will guide, nurture, encourage and quietly control. In the first few seconds he is in full control, and can set the scene. The conciliator throughout the meeting will use the basic skills of a meeting chairman, but without resorting to formal meeting phraseology or manner. As a general rule, the usual tools for informality can be used – jackets off, first names and open body language. As with all general rules, the exceptions are important. Often the NHS professionals will not want patients to use their first names. Equally often, the patients may not want to address a consultant surgeon as 'Fred'. Where the conciliator identifies that these factors apply, he must also use the more formal form of address, but with a casual, informal edge to his voice.

A successful outcome may take the full time of the meeting to achieve. On the other hand, unfortunately, it is possible to ensure failure within the first few seconds. In all situations, it is a basic rule of life that nobody gets a second chance to make a first impression. Even though the parties to the conciliation meeting may have met many times before, the first impression created at this meeting can set the tone for the whole proceedings. If the instant reaction of the parties to each other, and to the conciliator, is very strongly negative, then the outcome will probably be negative. If the first reaction is positive, there is a fair chance of a positive outcome. Body language is the key to a successful start, and the conciliator is only in a position to control his own body language. Open body language by the conciliator, and positive responses to the body language displayed by the parties is the key to first impression success.

Careful judgement is needed to manage this period of opening the joint 'chat' prior to the identifiable start of the meeting. In some situations, it will be evident from the signals received from one or both parties that a fast start to controlled discussion is required. In other situations, a prolonged standing chat over coffee may be useful. Again the clues will come mainly from body language. If the parties are reacting positively to each other, a few extra minutes of casual chat may prepare the ground for a positive opening. If the parties are reacting in a clearly formal manner to each other, then it will be wise to settle them down quickly to the controlled discussion. In some situations the reactions will be less specific. If the reactions are mixed, the conciliator may decide to use his own body language and other communication skills to attempt to move the parties from their indecisive start to a positive mode. Only a conciliator who is able to control both his sending and receiving body language should attempt this.

Once the parties are sitting comfortably and ready to start the discussion proper, the conciliator adopts the role of a conciliatory chairman. He will guide the discussion, summarize at relevant points, and help the parties to recognize their own changes in position. The conciliator can logically control the opening totally. The best opening format will be to summarize the situation which has developed since his own involvement. This means starting with the two stories as told to him by the parties. Whilst this will include their own recall of the involvement of other parties such as complaints managers, it will not include the opinions of those third parties unless the conciliator can use those third party opinions to illustrate agreement reached to date. The objective of the conciliator's introductory summary is to illustrate progress made already, and highlight the small amount of movement needed, or the low number of outstanding points of disagreement. The conciliator can achieve this by recalling a large number of points on which agreement has been reached, or by simply spending more time on the agreement achieved than on the outstanding disagreement. At all costs, the conciliator must illustrate that as some agreement has already been achieved at the pre-meetings, it is possible to achieve full agreement at this meeting. Once this opening is complete, the conciliator will have less direct control over proceedings. He should allow a wide discussion and will probably expect that one or both parties will start by revisiting points on which prior agreement has been achieved. In doing this the parties will be openly attempting to bolster their position as agreeable, flexible, helpful parties. Whilst so doing, they may actually be covertly attempting to strengthen an inflexible position on the outstanding issues. The conciliator must take each point of movement put forward by the party, and illustrate it as a point of mutual flexibility, thus undermining any attempt to adopt rigid positions. It is quite usual for the parties to attempt to use the first few minutes of discussion to strengthen their adopted positions. It is, therefore, at this stage that the conciliator can use his skills to constantly illustrate that movement has taken place, is taking place, and will take place.

The conciliator must also ensure that only facts and opinions are discussed at this early stage. If he allows attitudes to become dominant, movement by the parties is likely to cease. The techniques for keeping attitudes out include changing the subject, specifically setting the point aside for later, ignoring it, or using controlled body language to silence the person raising the item. All or any of these techniques can work. Attitudes, however, can be so dominant in a person's mind that they will not be easily set aside. The conciliator having analysed the total issue into facts, opinions and attitudes before the meeting, should be able to spot an attitude in its earliest stage of introduction and 'kill' it before it is expressed in full (Case Study 9).

Case Study 9

A conciliator was attempting to help a mental health trust and the family of a patient to reach agreement over the only real outstanding issue. This was an allegation by the family that they had not been involved in, or agreed to, the post-discharge care plan. The trust claimed that two members of the family had been present at the main planning meeting, but had failed to turn up at the final meeting when only minor adjustments were made. In the pre-meetings, the conciliator had, among other items, gained movement from the family insofar as they accepted that they had participated in a meeting, that they had received a very short notice invitation to the final meeting and that they were content with the majority of the plan content. The trust had 'moved' in confirming that only one day's notice was given for the final meeting, and that one substantial change had been made at the final meeting, plus a couple of minor adjustments. The conciliator had categorized the trust view of the family refusal to accept the major change as 'attitude'. He did this as a result of a number of clues, including the use of the word 'bigoted' by the trust medical director to describe the rejection. After introductions the conciliator guided detailed discussion around and about the minor changes for 15 minutes. He then helped the family to introduce the question 'why?' to the major change. In effect, the final discharge plan meeting was then re-run for 20 minutes, discussing the factors leading to the change, but not the change itself. After this time the family actually suggested an inclusion in the plan which was, in effect, the original major change differently worded. The parties accepted the 'new' plan, and parted in agreement. The failure to invite in time and/or attend the final meeting was basically ignored, and caused no further difficulties, and conciliation was achieved. This case illustrates that it is possible for a conciliator to overcome an attitude by simply by-passing it. The technique is not guaranteed success, but attempting it rarely causes any additional problems.

By the technique of controlling the topics discussed, and limiting them to facts and opinions, the conciliator should be able to help the parties to achieve further movement and gain agreement on a point, no matter how small. By his own strong and positive reaction to the new agreement, particularly through the further use of body language, he must attempt to infect the parties with his own enthusiasm for the agreement. Positive actions and positive reactions are the key tool to achieve an agreement through conciliation.

The conciliator's skill during the meeting is to observe, note and use a series of apparently insignificant points of communication by the parties.

The main techniques are the use of listening skills and body language, which are discussed in depth in the following passages. 'Clues' to movement do occur regularly throughout the meeting. Some of them are:

- A change of wording – A party may start by using a phrase such as 'I know it was at 10.00 a.m.'. If this changes to 'it was at about 10.00 a.m.' or 'it was at 10.00 a.m.', then movement is beginning. The first signals the start of flexibility, the second indicates a firming of position. The changes of phrase are not necessarily so subtle. In some cases the change may be to 'it was certainly in the morning', suggesting that major change has occurred.
- A change of direction – One of the parties may cease to speak to the conciliator, and start to address the other party direct. This is a clear change, and may not involve new language. The conciliator will need to regard body language associated with the change. If the body language becomes more 'open' between the parties, this suggests positive movement. If the body language becomes aggressive, this indicates a strengthening of adopted position(s).
- Introductory phrases – As each person starts to speak, they will use an introduction of some sort. Phrases such as 'my fair and reasonable view is that ...' usually precede an attitude. The conciliator needs to be very careful to control the statement which follows such a starter. Another introductory phrase which usually precedes a negative point is 'with respect to Mr Brown, ...'. Generally this is the introduction to telling Mr Brown that he is wrong, often without any sound foundation beyond attitude. Many negative introductions can be used. 'It is a fact ...' usually precedes an opinion without sound base. 'You will of course, accept that ...' almost always starts a point that will be rejected. 'Most reasonable people ...' is a very good way of trying to prove the other side is unreasonable. With all of these the conciliator's job is to clarify and minimize the negative effect of the words. Summarizing, asking for objective proof, ignoring, changing the subject and reacting positively are all tools the conciliator can use.

Positive introductory phrases will also occur. 'I accept that ....' shows positive movement. 'You may have a point ...' is clearly useful. 'Are you saying that ...' really depends upon what follows, but clearly indicates that the party who is using the phrase is thinking about the point. Even negative thinking is better than outright rejection. Any opener with one of Rudyard Kipling's six honest serving men is seeking information, and as such is positive. What, why, when, how, where, who, were Kipling's original six. 'Which' is another information-seeking opener. When a party uses such an open question as their introduction, the conciliator must seize upon the opportunity to promote positive discussion and movement.

Other openers indicating positive movement include 'that is a good point....', 'thank you for ....', 'let's move on ....', 'it is time to change ...', 'can you explain ....'. In fact, any opener that signifies acceptance, change, flexibility, information seeking or a desire to move forward is an open invitation to the conciliator to encourage further movement.

If the conciliator has prepared a staged plan, based on the identified minimum and ideal expectations of the parties, he should also be able to estimate the response of each party to movement by the other. The degree of movement, and the predictability of the response, will give the conciliator clear indications of progress against his original plan as the joint meeting develops. One very important point during such movements is that the egos of the parties must not be 'injured' by any action of the conciliator or the other party. Loss of face will cause a party to reject a solution that earlier indications might have suggested would be accepted. No one likes to have his feelings hurt, or to be humiliated in public. The individual's perception of humiliation varies from person to person, and the conciliator must be very sensitive to human feelings.

In handling these positive moves, and overcoming negative movement, the conciliator has to use his own communication skill and technique to develop the positive movement to a point of agreement. These include regular, positive summary of the points agreed to date, frequent encouragement of the less communicative persons, and recognition of individual and group contribution. In fact, all the standard techniques of a good chairman and communicator will be used to move the parties towards agreement.

There is one trap the conciliator must avoid; this is called the inspiration trap. Simply because the conciliator is a lay person, and is comparatively objective, he is likely to spot the obvious solution first. Usually this will be a simple compromise which, the conciliator feels, any reasonable person will accept. The conciliator, on seeing his solution, will be tempted to tell the parties exactly how to resolve their differences. This would be moving from conciliation to arbitration. The conciliator must avoid the temptation. The mediator, on the other hand, being an expert, can move cautiously but positively towards his solution.

The conciliator needs to use the power of suggestion to ensure that one party, or in a state of perfection both parties, actually spots and suggests the solution themselves. In conciliation there is no compulsion on the parties to stick to the agreement reached. The parties are most likely to stick with a solution which they 'own'. A solution which is perceived as 'imposed' by the conciliator may not survive the parties leaving the room. If the parties believe that they have invented and developed the solution themselves, they are very likely to stay with it. The technique to ensure that the parties spot the obvious is called seeding. The conciliator takes a small point from one or other of the parties and restates it in a minor variation which hints at the ideal solution, but does not state it. He then does exactly the same with a point from the other party. Having sown the seed he then sits back and lets discussion proceed. The conciliator may need to 'seed' the solution three or four times before the parties have their own inspiration. The conciliator will often find that the parties produce the solution in small parts. If this occurs, he should react positively, either verbally or with body language, to reinforce the positive movement. Eventually, it should be possible to bring the parties to their own version of the obvious solution, and then to accept it.

Now comes the end of the meeting. Some meeting chairmen actually find the end of a meeting to be the most difficult bit. Effectively conciliation is ended as soon as the parties have reached agreement. If a serious matter of attitude is involved, the conciliator needs to recognize that conciliation is achieved when all other matters have been agreed, and only the attitude matter is outstanding. The attitude point cannot be settled by movement on the part of the person holding the attitude. The very nature of attitude is such that it is not based on any foundation which is capable of change. Thus, if the other party will move, or accept the right of the first party to hold the attitude, then that point can be left out of the agreement on an 'agree to differ' basis. As will be seen later, absolute and diametrically opposed attitudes virtually rule out the possibility of successful conciliation.

Once the conciliator has decided that agreement is achieved, or that no further benefit will come from continuing, he must decide to bring the meeting to an end. The parties may benefit from a few minutes of chat, rather like the opening coffee chat. In fact a cup of coffee may be a good closing device. In any event, the conciliator must summarize the agreement(s) reached. He will, if necessary, specify any areas of non-agreement. As the agreement is not binding, the conciliator must take all the necessary steps to ensure that the parties do not back down on their given word – summarizing helps. A carefully composed and distributed written confirmation may be perceived by the parties as conferring a legally binding status on the agreement. Many people simply believe that once something is in black and white it has to be adhered to. The conciliator can use this human belief to advantage. If the facility is available, an instant written confirmation signed by both parties and the conciliator to take away from the meeting could be very useful. As a second string, the conciliator may agree to confirm the agreement in writing. If he does so, it must be very fast and preferably posted first class the same day.

7

The processes of conciliation and mediation

The process of conciliation is well known to most of us. Within the family, workplace, social circle etc. we routinely find ourselves positioned between two parties in some sort of disagreement. When this occurs, we have to make a decision. Basically there are three options: we can decide to take sides; we can turn our back and walk away; or we can act as an 'honest broker' to help the two sides resolve their dispute.

When such a domestic crisis occurs, we frequently take sides. If everybody takes sides then the dispute tends to grow. Eventually, the dispute will either fade away, or somebody will initiate an action which gets the two sides talking.

In conciliation within a complaints procedure, the options to take sides or walk away do not exist. The conciliator must act as the 'honest broker' and attempt not only to get the two sides communicating, but to assist and guide that communication with the objective of achieving an acceptable settlement of the dispute.

The basic principle involved in conciliation is for an independent third party to attempt to resolve an apparently inconsolable difference between two parties to a level accepted by both parties as a reasonable resolution of the conflict. In some cases there may be more than two parties involved; usually this would be a case of two of the parties being in some form of agreement, with a third party at loggerheads with the first two. It is possible for even more complicated situations to be placed before a conciliator. In one case, the complaint involved a GP, an ambulance trust, two acute hospital trusts, a community health care trust and the local authority social services department. The health authority manager of complaints acted as conciliator, and was accepted as neutral as the heath authority itself was not directly involved. The conciliation required numerous telephone conversations, and was successfully concluded with a two-hour meeting attended by over 20 people.

The conciliator may decide that he needs to carry out some investigation after the initial meetings with the parties. If a conciliator does carry out such investigation it should be only to the extent needed to obtain facts for use in conciliation. It is not the conciliator's role to re-investigate the issue of the complaint. The mediator will certainly want to see all the relevant medical notes at an early stage.

Conciliation as a technique for formal use within businesses and other organizations is a comparatively new development and very little help with the process is available in the form of training or printed guidelines. Most of the available works concern either conciliation in international disputes (often summaries of United Nations activities), or summaries of industrial disputes (often published by the UK Advisory, Conciliation and Arbitration Service [ACAS]).

The conciliator will adopt the non-directive approach, whilst the mediator will be clearly directive. The directive approach consists of the mediator being an 'expert' in his/her field. The mediator can then direct the conversation between the parties, using his/her expertise to respond to points raised by both parties in an appropriate way. The non-directive conciliator, on the other hand, will act exclusively as a summarizer, persuader, key point identifier, pacifier etc., without expressing clear opinions or views.

Every conciliation is unique, so the script cannot be written in advance. There are, however, a number of steps that often occur. The steps which will normally occur in either conciliation or mediation are laid out in Box 7.1. This process is also summarized as a flow chart in Appendix 1.

Box 7.1 THE CONCILIATION PROCESS

- Party A tell the conciliator their story.
- Party B tell the conciliator their story.
- The conciliator summarizes the party A story back to party A.
- The conciliator summarizes the party B story back to party B.
- The conciliator analyses both stories to find any common ground or points of agreement, and any points of clear disagreement.
- The conciliator divides the above points into facts, opinions, attitudes.
- The conciliator checks the 'facts' which are disputed to identify the true facts.
- The conciliator compares the opinions to find reasonable interpretations of both sides' opinions which develop further common ground.
- The conciliator summarizes his 'common ground' of party A's story to party A.
- The conciliator summarizes his 'common ground' of party B's story to party B.
- The conciliator listens to the responses of both parties to confirm common ground.
- The conciliator summarizes party A's total 'common ground' to party B.
- The conciliator summarizes party B's total 'common ground' to party A.

Box 7.1: *continued*

- The conciliator gains agreement of both parties to all common ground.
- The conciliator discusses the disputed facts with the two parties, introduces his factual checks and gains the agreement of both parties to the actual facts. It is important to start a process of 'movement' based on disputed facts.

The conciliator has now reduced the disagreement to opinions and attitudes. Thus far the conciliator has probably not sought to bring the two parties together. In effect, conciliation is about to commence. In a 'normal' situation, the disagreement is now isolated to a very clear set of issues, usually very low in number, often very strongly felt.

- The conciliator separates the opinions from the attitudes.
- The conciliator discusses the opinions of party A with party B.
- The conciliator discusses the opinions of party B with party A.
- The conciliator discusses the responses of party A with party B.
- The conciliator discusses the responses of party B with party A.

The conciliator *must* get each party to 'move' on an opinion at this stage

- The conciliator gains agreement from both parties that the 'other side' has a basis for their opinion.
- The conciliator invites the parties to meet to discuss their differing opinions under his/her chairmanship, with the objective to move the differences of opinion closer together and maximize agreement.
- On obtaining an acceptable level of agreement on opinions, the conciliator introduces the attitudes, and attempts to achieve agreement to the right of the other party to their thoughts, without attempting to change attitude.
- The conciliator then attempts to summarize the issues, highlighting agreements and specifying points of difference, and gains agreement that the latter will not be resolved but can be left as acknowledged by the other party.
- The conciliator ensures that the parties accept the agreed situation and arranges appropriate confirmation. The conciliator attempts to ensure that the parties accept the agreement as final, but has no power to make it binding.

In mediation cases it is often a good idea to bring the two parties together briefly at the start of the process to identify clear points of difference. The parties may then be separated to conduct the stages listed above, before being brought together again at the end to achieve agreement. A very experienced mediator may actually conduct the whole process in one meeting, without separating the parties. This strategy can greatly reduce the time taken, but does carry a greater risk of failure. In some instances a very experienced conciliator may also adopt this one meeting process, but the risks involved are even greater than in mediation.

There is no standard formula for calculating the time necessary to achieve conciliation or mediation. Generally speaking the time for an NHS complaint conciliation is expected to be measured in hours rather than minutes or days; mediation of a medical nature should take less time on average than conciliation.

The check list in Appendix 2 may be useful when preparing to conciliate or mediate.

8

Listening techniques

Listening is very simple really, it is just one more communication technique. We are all taught communication techniques at some stage in our lives. We are usually taught the skill of spoken language first, as Mum or Dad talk to us parrot fashion until we say our first word, then the process of saying and understanding words continues through our whole life. The next stage of communication comes in the form of writing and then reading. Today most working people are also taught the electronic communication skills such as telephone techniques, fax, electronic mail etc. Salesmen are taught to hear buying signals. But very few of us are taught to listen. For many of us, our lifetime listening skills training consists of an adult saying to us 'little children were meant to be seen but not heard, so shut up and listen!!'. This is bad advice, on two counts. First, we are meant to communicate, which must involve a two-way transaction. Second, if we shut up, we are not listening actively.

There is a distinct difference between hearing and listening. Hearing is the process or power of hearing sound. To listen is to pay attention in order to hear. Apart from those who suffer from hearing impairment, most of us can perceive sounds. We can even be selective in the sounds that we hear. People who work on or close to airports can conduct a meeting during the take off and landing of aircraft without raising their voices. To an occasional visitor it seems impossible, but the locals' hearing ability has cut out the extraneous noise. We all do this, and it can affect our ability to listen. On our own territory, we are so used to the noise, or to the silence, that we ignore it in conversation. To listen, we must recognize that our visitors will hear the noise of the office, or traffic, or wildlife, and that it will interfere with their ability to communicate.

There are many different reasons to listen. Many people like to listen to their favourite music. A good technique for this is to close the eyes and lie back. This passive listening technique will not work when listening to a person who is talking to you. When listening to a good play or soap on the radio or television, a very great deal is left to one's own imagination, and the way we interpret such entertainment varies from person to person. This is exactly as it should be, but when a person is telling us about a problem, we must listen so that we understand exactly what the perceived problem is in the mind of the speaker. Our own interpretation is not relevant. Our own views, opinions and emotions need to be set aside and the views, opinions and emotions of the speaker need to be understood. This is the listening technique that will be discussed in this chapter. It is normally described as 'active listening'. Active listening not only requires that we hear what is said, but also that we impress upon the speaker that we are, indeed, hearing, understanding and accepting what he is saying.

For active listening, human beings are equipped with a number of tools. This chapter will discuss each of those tools in turn. The tools are:

- The eyes – used to make eye contact during listening. Many aspects of eye contact are also covered in Chapter 9.
- The mouth – Contrary to some popular belief, it is quite wrong to stay silent during active listening.
- The body, fully described in Chapter 9, is used as an important part of the process of listening.
- Physical appearance – This is a major part of the first impression, and there is no second chance.
- Questions – To ask for more information or clarification is a clear part of active listening.
- The brain – Analysing, summarizing and reflecting the points stated by the speaker is an active part of the listening process.
- The voice – The speaker's voice will vary in tone: recognition of the meanings of tone of voice is very useful as part of active listening.
- The hands – To make notes of the key points so that the communication can be confirmed and agreed. This is a key part of active listening.
- Time – Conciliation and listening both demand the commitment of some time.
- The ears – Self-evident perhaps, but unless a listener opens his ears and hears what is said, listening cannot occur.

Let us start with the eyes. 'Look at me when I am talking to you' is a common comment by talkers. The question is, exactly where do we look to listen? Direct eye contact, absolute staring at the eyes of the other person, is not the answer as this is over-aggressive. Neither is it right to look near the eyes. If one person looks just to the side of the speaker's head, the impression given is that no listening is taking place at all. In fact, the speaker will actually become disconcerted. The speaker may think that something more important is happening behind him. He may even stop speaking, and look round to see what is going on. Listening has been disturbed, possibly even the relationship between speaker and listener may have been damaged. A total failure to make any eye contact at all is also the antithesis of good listening. The speaker will not continue for very long if the 'listener' is constantly looking down at his feet, or up in the air. So what is good eye contact for listening? The answer is to make and break eye contact frequently, regularly and appropriately. Some call this a glancing technique: make contact, hold it briefly, and break it. If the make and break can be synchronized with points the speaker believes are important, this is capable in its own right of convincing the speaker that they are being properly listened to. Eye contact should be made at least at 20-second intervals, and each contact held for about three to ten seconds. In some situations this is quite easy to achieve. For a receptionist, for example, who is making notes, it is easy to make eye contact, break away, make a note, and return to eye contact. The conciliator should be making notes as part of the active listening technique, and use the same movement. If it is felt necessary to confirm good eye contact, this can be done by observing people in a restaurant or bar. Try to measure the amount of eye contact that people make with each other during their private conversations. Then try to guess the relationship of the people in those conversations. There will probably be pairs looking languidly into each other's eyes for extended periods: these will be classified as new lovers. There will be couples where one stares at the other, and the second person looks away. These will be classified as a dominant and passive pair. There will be those whose whole body declares that they are making an important point, and the listener will be looking at their eyes at that moment.

In this experiment, it is also a good idea to note where the eyes of each party are directed when they are not looking at their partner's eyes. It is very unlikely that they will make any eye contact with the restaurant staff, unless they want service. In fact, people will discuss their most intimate secrets in the hearing of receptionists, waiters, bar staff, taxi drivers and other service providers, and because they make no eye contact with those people, they will believe that the staff cannot hear, or understand, what they are saying. So powerful are the eyes in listening, that the eyes alone can 'hear', or ignore, speech almost unaided.

Notice also that many eyes will turn to a new event. If a new person walks into the room, everybody will glance at him. If a waiter drops a plate, all eyes turn in that direction. Whilst the eyes are turned away, no listening takes place. This is a secondary message for the use of the eyes in listening. If the eyes are distracted, they switch off the ears. Thus, the conciliator must take all reasonable steps to ensure that neither he nor the parties are distracted during communication. The room should be set up, for example, with the conciliator controlling the view through the window. Then, if a distraction to the eyes occurs outside, the conciliator can control its effect on the listening process, the easy way being to mention it and dismiss it. This will enable all those in the room to resume active listening. As the eyes are one of the primary tools of listening, it is wise to be well aware of their importance.

Now let us look at the use of the mouth. The mouth forms the words that have to be heard. Most people can lip read to some extent. When a footballer utters foul language in the middle of the pitch, the television viewer cannot hear the words but has no doubt about the words used.

Using the eyes to watch the speaker's mouth when not in eye contact can aid listening. But the listener's mouth has a much more pro-active role to play in listening. Total silence during listening is not helpful. The speaker expects to hear some clear acknowledgement that they have been heard. The 'grunting' technique comes into its own here. Throat noises such as 'ahah', 'ummh', 'yeah' can be very comforting to the speaker, provided they come at the right moments. This becomes a self-funding technique, as the only way to ensure that the grunts are well timed, is to open the ears and listen. A grunting technique, synchronized with body language such as head nodding, eyebrow raising and eye contact, is a very powerful active listening tool. In fact, if the conciliator uses nothing else from this book but this combination, the return on investment will be well worthwhile. The mouth is also used to express the questions and reflection discussed later in this chapter.

The mouth could also be said to be the source of silence. A period of silence when the speaker is expecting to hear a comment can often gain extra information. Commonly called the pregnant pause, staying silent with neutral body language for ten seconds after the speaker has stopped is a very useful tool for the active listener. This is particularly useful to seek expansion on a complex opinion, or to start checking on a possible untruth.

The whole body can be used to listen. In particular, the arms, face, hands and eyes can be used to impress upon the speaker that he is being listened to. The techniques of body language are discussed at length in the next chapter, but the point is made here that the body is a listening tool.

Physical appearance is part of the listening process. The major effect of physical appearance is the first impression which the conciliator makes on the parties, and vice versa. Whenever one human being sees another for the first time, he forms an opinion of that person. That opinion goes way beyond assessing wealth or class. The observer will decide on the profession, the personality, the honesty, the friendliness, the sex appeal and many other factors all based on the first impression which is a combination of appearance and body language. Most people have experienced the situation where a person enters the room, and all conversation stops. Everybody present looks at the new arrival and makes an assessment. Many people are reluctant to go out alone to a bar or restaurant because of this phenomenon.

The conciliator needs to be aware of this phenomenon. He will gain an impression of the parties on first meeting, or even on first telephone conversation. The conciliator must be able to limit the effect this has on his subsequent dealings with the party. The conciliator must also be aware of the first impression his own appearance will create. The complainant, or the professional, will not try to communicate with a conciliator who has made a seriously bad first impression. Thus appearance is a part of listening: you cannot listen if nobody talks to you. It is not easy to control some aspects of appearance. If the conciliator is exceptionally short or tall, fat or thin then he should take such steps as are possible to minimize negative effects. The effect of height, for example, is minimized by sitting down. The clothing worn is totally controllable. In most cases the conciliator will be expected to be 'smart and business like'. This is fairly easy to achieve: it simply means neutral clothing, nothing outlandish or extreme. There is a small need here to refer back to the brain usage – if the conciliator has a strong opinion or attitude that jeans and sweat shirt should be accepted as business clothing, then he will need to overcome his own thoughts and accept the majority view of business clothing.

Asking questions is part of listening. To actively seek more information from the speaker is not interrupting, it is listening. The questions normally start with open questions. Any question starting with what, when, why, how, who, which or when is seeking to get a reply which gives broad information. If a party tells the conciliator that he was upset at the way in which a nurse dealt with his request, the conciliator might ask 'How did it upset you?' to get a full, and uncontrolled, mass of information. Alternatively 'How did the nurse respond?' will still gain wide information, but on a different aspect of the subject. The use of open questions is yet another very powerful tool for the active listener. It is sometimes a good listening technique to use a series of open questions. This can be particularly useful where the speaker is, or is becoming, aggressive. With aggressive people it is useful to extract every last detail, and gain agreement through reflection, before offering any response at all.

Specific questions are also useful in listening. Usually, the specific question is used to check or confirm a detail that has come from an open question. A specific question will usually elicit a short, but not superficial response. In the situation used above with the nurse, for example, after the open question a specific question might be 'Can you tell me any of the technical jargon the nurse used?'. With luck, this will give the conciliator some specific points to use with the nurse to gain movement in the conciliation process.

Once the conciliator has gained all the information he needs, or is able to elicit, it may be necessary to use a closed question to finish the conversation. A closed question should receive a simple yes or no as the answer, and the effect is often to stop the speaker, without the speaker realizing that they have been stopped by another person's deliberate action. The closed question can be used also to check the details – 'I think that the points you have made are x, y and z. Am I correct?'

The active listener's brain needs to be in top gear throughout the process. It is said that the average human being is capable of concentrating for only a few seconds at a time. The conciliator must force himself to listen for several minutes at a time. This may well be done by stringing several shorter periods together. It may be that the conciliator can use his eye movement and body language deliberately to utilize a few milliseconds between bouts of listening. At the end of the day, the conciliator is listening for very small clues to movement by the parties and must not miss anything.

Quite often the party or parties will repeat their points several times. The listening conciliator can use these periods of repetition for two purposes. The first is to rest between bouts of concentration, deliberately and for a controlled, very short period. The second is to listen very intently for any change of emphasis in the second or subsequent telling. Any change of emphasis, perhaps just a substituted word, may be a hint of movement. It is also necessary to mention that precise repetition, without any change of wording or tone of voice, probably means that a rehearsed story is being told. If the story is rehearsed it may not be a true recall. Open questions thrown in at the middle of such a repetition can help to upset the rehearsed routine, and get closer to the real and current recall of the party.

The brain must also be used during listening to analyse the information coming from the party or parties. This is clearly easier during the pre-meetings stage when only one party is present. Note taking can help with the analysis. The conciliator has to constantly search through all the information coming from the party for clues to a solution, and for movement. Fortunately the human brain is capable of dual function. Any person who can read a newspaper whilst watching television, or talk to a friend in the bar whilst watching an attractive person walk by, has this dual function capability. A little mind training, done simply by practice, can sharpen the brain considerably to be more expert at multiple thought usage.

One technique of brain usage is particularly important for the conciliator. The need to analyse the issues into opinions, attitudes and facts has been stated many times. The conciliator is also a human being. He has his own opinions and attitudes. The conciliator may be called upon to deal with persons of a type he has not experienced before. NHS complainants are not all middle class, professional, family men with standard ethical and moral standards. The conciliator may need to help resolve a case involving a single parent with a criminal background. The conciliator's own views of the sanctity of marriage and the lawless state of the country may exist, but the conciliator has to be able to use his own brain to recognize that his clients' values are different and valid, and they also exist. In some cases the very nub of the dispute may be a difference in such attitudes or values. The conciliator may feel that he sympathizes with one party on that score. Even so, the conciliator must remain neutral, a clear case of mind control. The key to this is to keep the conciliation objective clearly at the front of the mind. The objective is to resolve the problem by helping the parties to reach agreement through discussion, nothing more, nothing less. Any agreement, no matter how illogical, is the objective.

Another aspect of the effect of the brain on listening is the feelings, emotions and moods of the listener and the parties. Ideally there would be no emotion and everything would be a matter of logic and objectivity. Unfortunately, all the people involved are human beings who are emotional animals. People cry when a character in a TV soap is 'killed off'. There is no logic to such a reaction, everybody knows that actors are playing a part, but we react emotionally. If this reaction to unreal situations occurs, then clearly the parties will have emotional reactions to events that concern them. In some cases complainants will be a bereaved family. Where the deceased is a young family member, emotions will be high. It is a good idea for the conciliator to be aware of the stages of bereavement which occur, as they may well affect his handling of a conciliation communication. The listener's job is to control his own moods and emotions, whilst recognizing the moods of the parties.

The tone of voice is a tool supplied by the speaker. Try saying the following sentence with the emphasis moving from word to word, 'I think that you are a wonderful person'. It is possible purely by transfer of emphasis to change the meaning from the basic written words to 'I hate you'. By varying the emphasis more, and by introducing strength to the voice at different points, the same phrase can move from a great compliment to a sexual innuendo. The active listener must listen for tone of voice. In a book it is difficult to describe the subtle changes which take place in a speaker's voice. The conciliator will need to apply his own experience of life to the interpretation of signals contained in tone of voice. One very good exercise is to video-record a subtitled film in a foreign language which the listener does not understand. Play part of the video and listen with the eyes shut or the back turned. Remember the impression you get purely from the voice tone. Then play the same piece again, reading the subtitles. There is a very high probability that the listener will have judged the mood correctly. In the second viewing, with the advantage of body language added, the listener may even understand the gist of what is said without understanding a word that is spoken. This is the total power of non-verbal communication.

Taking notes is a clear part of listening. To the speaker it implies that he is being taken seriously. For the listener it gives a fairly objective recall of the conversation. Absolute recall may be achieved by the use of a tape recorder, but this is often taken as intimidating by the parties and can lead to communication breakdown. Taking notes during a conversation, whilst also analysing, observing body language, making eye contact etc., requires some practice. This is particularly true if the best setting of a comfortable armchair has been used for the meetings. Taking notes on one's knee, with a floppy piece of paper can be very difficult. The techniques used vary from person to person. Preparation is the key to success. Prepare the media to be used and the format to be used.

One useful tool for note taking in this situation is to carry small cards. Postcards or kardex-type cards are useful. They are a convenient size and they have their own rigidity to help with the note taking. An alternative is to carry a clip board. Clip boards do come in a variety of sizes, the most common is A4 or foolscap. Smaller boards can be found or made. A piece of stiff cardboard cut to size with a bulldog clip can do very nicely. A less formal approach is to carry a magazine and some A4 paper in the briefcase or handbag. The magazine provides an informal way of introducing note-taking, as well as a stiff backing for the paper. Shorthand pads, notebooks, organizer-type diaries are all possible tools for note taking.

The format is also very much a matter of taste. The majority of people simply make a list of points chronologically as they are raised by the speaker. A conciliator might want to prepare a multi-column format where he can make his lists from the different parties alongside each other, thus giving him instant analysis but difficulty in locating the place to write points from second or subsequent parties. Some people like to use the newish 'mind map' style of note taking. Basically this method consists of starting with a central note, and 'mapping' thought in logical or natural groups around the central theme. For those who are practised in the use of mind maps it provides an easy way of making similar and easily comparable notes with all parties.

Time is needed to listen actively: not necessarily a great deal of time, but certainly enough to allow the speaker to express all his views, opinions and emotions on the topic in question. A good listener will not rush the speaker. Listening requires two parties, a sender and a receiver. Both must be able to devote enough time to the communication to enable the sender to articulate his thoughts and for the receiver to hear, understand and interpret those thoughts. The receiver then needs sufficient time to confirm with the sender that he has understood and interpreted something very close to the original meaning and belief of the sender. At the same time, a conciliator will not want to waste anybody's time. The speaker will often tend to get into a round of multiple repetition of the same story. This is a point at which the listener can use closing techniques to make the listening process time efficient. The active listener must achieve a balance between devoting the time perceived as needed by the parties, and the commitment of resources.

Finally we consider the ears. It may seem strange to leave the ears to last, but in reality the ears are the easiest of all the tools to recognize and use. The ears are nothing more than a channel to take the words of the speaker from the speaker's mouth to the listener's brain. Unfortunately the ears are easily switched off or closed. This happens particularly if the eyes are distracted. It may sound daft to say it, but whilst we can easily close our ears, we cannot close our eyes. In human communication terms this is very true. It is widely accepted that 80% of the information stored in our brain came via the eyes, 17% via the ears and the balance through all the other senses. Thus the brain is set up to give priority to information gained through sight. The active listener must train his ears to work and mentally record every meaning expressed.

Finally, it is necessary to record the conciliator's role in ensuring that the parties use active listening skills. It is very unlikely that the parties will have been trained to use active listening. It is also very likely that one or both parties will have the common communication barrier of hearing what they want to hear, rather than what is said. To overcome these barriers to communication, the conciliator will need to use his own high-level communication skills and the techniques of a first-class chairman at all meetings and discussions.

9

Using body language

Body language is an odd thing. We all speak and understand it. Devotees of body language declare that over 85% of face-to-face communication between human beings is 'non-verbal'. Debunkers believe that it is a load of rubbish, and that the spoken and written word is the sole communicator.

For a conciliator, it is wise to recognize that all people send 'signals' through things such as facial expression, body posture and gestures. Even the most sceptical will accept that an angry person can be spotted at a great distance by his stance and movement (Figure 9.1). Everybody prefers a smiling face (Figure 9.2) to a grimace (Figure 9.3). This chapter attempts to detail some of the more simple aspects of body language which a conciliator may find useful in his work.

Before looking at the details of body language it is essential to give a warning of the effects of culture. The suggestions in this chapter are safe to use when in a meeting of any sort with people who are from essentially a modern, western cultural base. Major differences do occur when dealing with people from other cultures. There are even some differences within a comparatively small area such as Europe. In the UK, for example, 'thumbs

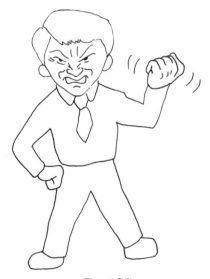

Figure 9.1

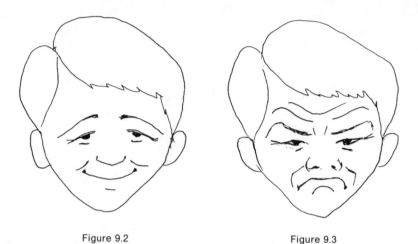

Figure 9.2   Figure 9.3

up' is a sign of a good result. In Greece the same sign is a serious insult. The differences within Europe, North America, Australia etc. are, however, generally minor in nature.

When it comes to other cultures the differences become quite major. In many Eastern cultures, for example, eye contact has very specific rules. One example is the caste system, where a lower caste person may not look in the eye of a higher caste person. Another example is that, in some countries, women may not look men in the eye. Arabs stand very close together when conversing, and even use the sense of smell as part of listening. This can result in quite a comical situation when, for example, an American and an Arab attempt to converse. The Arab constantly moves closer to the American, the American constantly backs off to achieve his 'space' requirement, and the two pursue each other around the room. It is not possible within one chapter to detail all the cultural differences, indeed nobody has yet fully researched the subject. The conciliator needs to be aware that where there is a cultural difference, he must be cautious in interpreting and using body language.

The conciliator's role with body language is threefold. First he needs to be able to receive and recognize the messages sent by the parties. Second he needs to understand the messages he is sending himself. Third, and by far the most difficult, he needs to manage his own body language to send and receive deliberate messages, and to help the parties to communicate. This chapter will work its way through a number of aspects of body language, giving details of the messages contained and tips on ways to control those messages.

The face is a very important part of the body for the purposes of communication. The smile is virtually universal across all cultures, and carries a similar meaning. The smile is inherently positive. It is a friendly, happy expression used to indicate pleasure, amusement, welcome, help and a wide variety of desirable emotions. Peculiarly, the smile even works without the benefit of sight. Telephone sales people are trained to smile when on the telephone, because it gives a positive edge to the voice. For the conciliator, the ability to smile when a party makes a small movement will be very helpful in encouraging more movement, and in helping the other party to spot and accept the movement. Training to smile is at the easier end of controlling body language. The result has to be a natural looking, pleasant smile. The conciliator does not want to present a replica of the plastic smile shown by synchronized swimmers as they come out of the water. A sickly grin must also be avoided; the best smile for deliberate use has the mouth still closed, but a distinct widening of the lips and a general 'lightness' to the whole face. One way to train the smiling muscles is to make oneself smile when something negative is happening, preferably when one is alone. Try to make the face smile when there is bad news on the television. Try to hold the smile for as long as possible. Once this is accomplished, repeat the smile in front of a mirror. As soon as you are confident, try using your new deliberate smile on other people in non-threatening situations. Note the effect of your smile: if it works well a majority of people, even strangers, will smile back; they cannot help it, that is body language.

There are other facial expressions which the conciliator can use. The frown is a simple one to use deliberately: it indicates either anger or derision. Used very briefly it can convey to a party that they are not co-operating as well as the conciliator would wish. The frown is very easy to initiate, most of us can frown deliberately quite easily. It is more difficult to control an involuntary frown. The conciliator may need to prevent himself frowning when a party gives a negative response. Training oneself to avoid frowning is very difficult. The exercise recommended above to deliberately smile is the key. When watching bad news on TV, we normally find our facial expression has moved to the frown. The frown can be felt in a physical tightening of the brow. Usually on TV bad news is predictable a few seconds ahead. Try preventing the brow from tightening as the bad news starts. This can be a difficult task, but if it can be achieved, then a deliberate non-frown can be used with parties.

The use of parts of the face is another aspect of facial expression. A raising of the eyebrows can strengthen a pregnant pause when listening (Figure 9.4). A nod of the head is very encouraging and will help a reluctant party to communicate. Raising all the parts of the face (eyes, brow, upper lips) together (Figure 9.5) can indicate surprise. All of these are fairly easy to do deliberately.

Finally the poker player expression can be useful. Good poker players train themselves to show no reaction whatever on their face when they see their hand. In some situations the conciliator may find it useful to adopt the 'poker face' and give the party no clue at all as to his reaction. Again in front of the mirror is a good place to train for this.

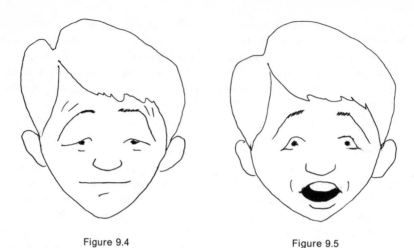

Figure 9.4   Figure 9.5

The eyes are also a key part of the body. The use of the eyes as a listening tool has already been discussed; however, they play a much more substantial role in communication. Eye contact can create or destroy relationships. Eye contact can establish faith, trust, love, hate etc. The really good politicians, evangelists, stage performers and others use eye contact to achieve their aims. One example is the way an evangelist makes eye contact with an audience of thousands. He roams his eyes over the audience in a set pattern, making contact with every person present regularly and frequently. The result is that five thousand people all believe that he was looking them personally in the eye all the time he was speaking, and they come forward as requested. Many researchers believe the eyes to be the most important single part of non-verbal communication.

Absolute eye contact, direct staring at each other's eyes (Figure 9.6), can trigger very violent reactions. If two people make such contact, the minimum result is that one has to look away, and the other 'wins'. In people with violent tendencies, eye contact is enough to start physical or verbal abuse. In a crowded room, two strangers can decide to become

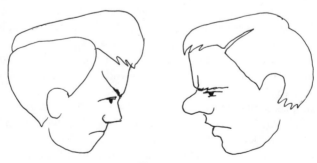

Figure 9.6

lovers, based on initial eye contact. Eye contact is constant among people in western society. People who are talking to each other usually make and break eye contact frequently, to reinforce communication. In a public place, people will try to make eye contact with persons they find attractive. This can start relationships if the contact is returned. If one person in a conversation diverts his eyes, looks around the room, watches other people, the other person in the conversation becomes frustrated at the lack of eye contact. Boredom is a clear message which we get from the eyes. People will adjust their whole body positions just to achieve better eye contact. When solicitors 'train' their clients to appear in court, they advise them to look at the magistrate when answering questions, not at the person who asked the question. Then they try to make the other side's witnesses look at them and not the magistrate whilst they carry out their own interrogation. All of these are indicators of the strength of eye contact as a communication tool. The conciliator needs to use eye contact, and the eyes in general, extensively.

In any conversation, initial eye contact has to be made to assure both parties that they have the attention of the other. The conciliator can easily establish eye contact with the other party. The conciliator needs to observe, in a joint meeting, to ensure that the two parties make direct eye contact. If they do not, he can use his own eye, and head, movement to encourage the parties to make contact. Encouragement is as far as he can go. If the parties absolutely refuse to make any eye contact at all, the conciliator will have to decide whether or not communication is feasible at the meeting. An adjournment to identify the cause of zero contact may be necessary.

Truthfulness is another aspect of communication for which the eyes can be helpful. Accomplished liars will have trained their eyes to hide their deceptions. The majority of people are not very skilful at telling untruths, and find it difficult to make eye contact whilst telling an untruth. Other body language factors taken with eye contact can give clear indications of the deceiver. The conciliator, if he suspects that a party is not being totally truthful from eye movement, should check the other signs. Good clues come from shuffling the feet, crossing and uncrossing legs, moving in the seat, touching the side of the neck or the nose, sweating, swallowing, fiddling with spectacles or other items in the hands (Figure 9.7). All of these may indicate that the person is uncomfortable with what they are saying. A combination of several clues is a strong indication, but one alone may simply mean, for example, that the chair is uncomfortable. The conciliator must spot the clues, and be aware that the other party will probably spot it even if he is not trained in body language. Most of us believe we can spot a liar.

A desire for information is communicated with the eyes. When a person makes eye contact as the other person stops speaking, more information is required. The signal may be negative or positive, but more information is required. The conciliator can spot this in a party, and encourage the first

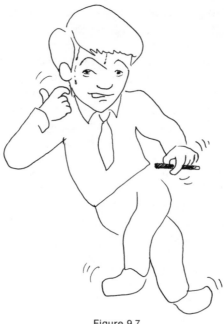

Figure 9.7

speaker to give more. Alternatively, the conciliator can use such eye contact with a pregnant pause to elicit more for himself.

The eyes can also be used to adopt positions. The dominant, or aggressive, position is the most common. This is done by the person who intends to dominate by 'staring out' the other party (Figure 9.6). The person attempting to dominate will also adopt a body position which makes him sit taller (Figure 9.8) than the other party, and the whole body will tend to be fairly rigid. If this occurs, it is very difficult for the conciliator to change things and therefore he needs to prevent dominance. The problem of dominance can only occur at the joint meeting. The signals should be spotted before that meeting starts, and the room laid out to minimize the effect. Ensuring that the dominant person does not sit directly face to face with the other party, that chairs are such that nobody can 'sit tall', positioning himself in a 'protective' chair can all reduce, but not eliminate, the opportunities for one person to dominate.

The pupils of the eyes are a little more difficult to observe, but they do give a very clear indication of a person's interest. Eckard Ess, a researcher into the subject, discovered that the pupils dilate or enlarge when a person looks at something which they find interesting. The pupils contract when uninteresting things occur. This appears to be a totally involuntary response, and is therefore a reliable indicator to the positive or negative reaction of each person present. The degree of dilation is directly proportional to the degree of positive response.

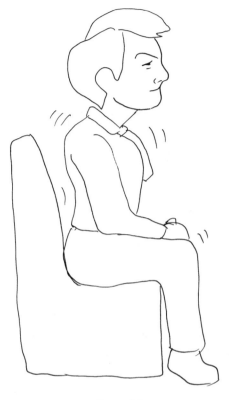

Figure 9.8

The head is logically the next part of the body to consider. The nodding head for yes, the shaking head for no are very clear and virtually cross all cultures. As an exercise in body language control try nodding the head whilst saying and meaning 'NO'. This is a very difficult trick to achieve, most people fail, and if you succeed the person with whom you are communicating will become very confused. This will demonstrate to you that absolute control of body language is very hard to achieve.

The use of the head nod and shake, however, is a simple and useful body language technique. When one party at the joint meeting has given a tiny indication of movement, try combining head nodding with eye contact. Your pupils will probably dilate because you are pleased at positive progress. Add some open body language, and there is a strong probability that the party concerned will instantly move further down the road of movement, without a spoken word from the conciliator. Equally, combining a mild head shake with eyes cast down and folded arms (Figure 9.9) will discourage a party from progressing further down a route the conciliator would prefer to avoid.

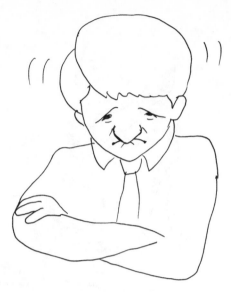

Figure 9.9

The head nod can carry a number of messages. It can signify acceptance, agreement, approval, encouragement, understanding, faith, belief, and a willingness to continue. A very enthusiastic nod indicates agreement to the point of full support. The conciliator will need to recognize the context of the nod, and its combination with other verbal and non-verbal communication to interpret and use the nod.

In all body language, reflecting or mirroring the body position (Figure 9.10) of the other person in the conversation indicates strong interest in

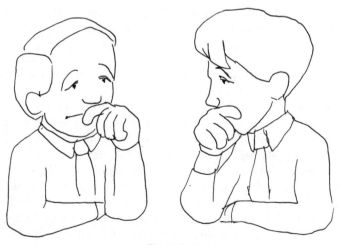

Figure 9.10

the other person. Quite often, in conversation, one of the parties will cock their head to one side. Generally speaking, cocking the head is an attempt to gain the attention of the other person. If the conciliator cocks his own head to mirror the party, then the party will believe that they have the whole attention of the conciliator. In the joint meeting, if one party cocks and the conciliator mirrors, there is a strong probability that the other party will join in and give the first party the attention they are seeking.

If a party rams his head forward from the shoulders (Figure 9.11), other parties will feel threatened. The forward thrust of the head is a very aggressive gesture. The conciliator can partially cancel the effect by instantly leaning has whole body backwards, adopting the fully open body position (Figure 9.12), and smiling at the threatened party. This will normally reduce the impact of the attempt at aggression. It is strange to note that a lesser tilt of the head, known as a court bow, is a specific sign of respect.

Most people will use their head movement to emphasize their point whilst speaking. We often nod our head whilst speaking to encourage others to agree with us. We use our head to indicate the person we are talking to, or talking about. We use our heads to encourage the others in a discussion to look in a certain direction. We also tend to move our heads closer as a sign of faith or confidentiality. The conciliator can train himself to use all of these points quite easily.

The whole body is more commonly used within body language when standing rather than when sitting, for obvious reasons. Impersonators, when preparing their act, study the whole body of the person they intend to impersonate. Stance, posture and gestures are all incorporated into the act. Next time an impersonator is on TV, try switching off the sound and

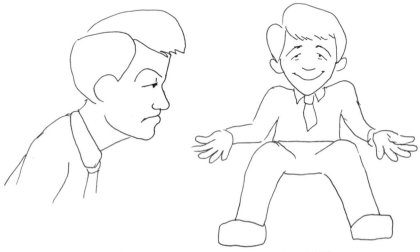

Figure 9.11   Figure 9.12

guessing which person is being copied. The fact that we can guess most of them correctly indicates just how much of an individual's communication comes from body language. A strong, upright body posture (Figure 9.13) indicates a positive, open, strong personality. This is a very easy posture to adopt at the point of first meeting. Before going through the door, stand tall, push the shoulders back, dry the palms of the hands, smile and then enter. The impact will be immediately clear. The same thing can be done in a chair at the joint meeting. If the conciliator sits tall, he will be accepted as a serious and positive influence on the meeting. To maintain the upright stance throughout a meeting of half an hour, however, requires discipline and training.

The extremes of full body language are the totally open and closed stances. The open and closed positions give a very clear indication to the other person that they are being listened to, or shut out. People very rarely adopt the absolute positions for extended periods. Indeed it could be said that the absolute closed position is to turn the back and adopt the foetal position. It is interesting that people who are mentally ill sometimes do exactly that, as a way of shutting out the world. The fully closed position (Figure 9.9) normally consists of folded arms, crossed legs, head cast down and eyes looking away or even closed. Partially closed is very common, and false signals can be given. The most common example of this is listening when standing, with the arms folded. Fortunately this is a comparatively easy position for the conciliator to train himself to avoid or adopt at will. As an exercise, the conciliator will inevitably find himself in some social gathering, standing with his arms folded whilst someone else is talking. Having noticed it, he can make himself gently unfold his arms,

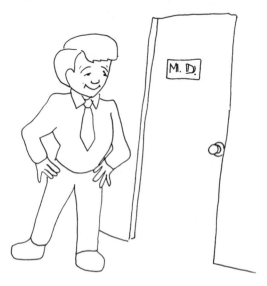

Figure 9.13

adopt the fully open position very briefly, then move to a neutral or partly open position. This is a simple exercise, but one that is very useful as a first attempt at body language control. Having successfully completed this exercise a few times, the conciliator ought to be able to avoid adopting the closed position unless he wants to convey a specific message.

The fully open position (Figure 9.14) is a little more complex to explain. It involves a positive facial expression, intermittent eye contact, upright body posture, arms extended downwards with the palms exposed to the other person, legs relaxed with the feet pointing outwards at an angle of 90° to each other. If the conciliator adopts this position, preferably in private, he will see that it is overall rather a silly way to stand for any length of time. The way to use the open position is to adopt it very briefly from time to time when it is necessary to convince the other person(s) that they have complete, open, honest, neutral attention from the conciliator. A partial open position, such as hands open in the lap when sitting down, can be usefully held for extended periods.

Whole body posture is a useful indicator of the extent of emotions indicated by other parts of body language. People who are depressed to the level of clinical illness routinely adopt a very stooped, submissive, non-communicative posture for extended periods. Indeed, people who have been seriously ill may not recover an upright positive stance for many years after the illness is ended or controlled. This is an extreme example, but is intended to illustrate the way in which body language is

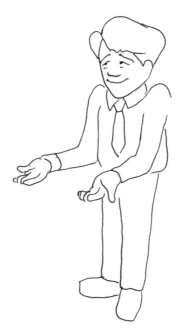

Figure 9.14

intensified in whole body stance. In the case of a positive acceptance of another person, for example by mirroring (Figure 9.10), if the person's body stance consists of a leaning towards each other, this indicates a very strong positive acceptance. Taken to extreme, this can indicate sexual attraction. The conciliator will, in the main, need to observe the whole body stance of the parties to gain clues to help with discussion and agreement. To a lesser extent, he may wish to use his own body to convince one or both parties that he is offering positive help.

Gestures are a normal part of our everyday communication, and the international spread of media and entertainment has made many gestures universal. Even so, there are gestures which have different meanings in different cultures. Gestures are used, sometimes deliberately, by people to assert attitudes or to convey specific messages. Shaking the fist is a common example of a deliberate gesture, hopefully one which will not enter the conciliator's field. One very common gesture is the praying motion (Figure 9.15). The hands are placed together, as in prayer, and lifted towards the chin. When sitting, this is often done with the elbows resting on the table. Generally, the praying motion accompanies a genuine wish to be believed, and indicates sincerity. The conciliator can train himself to use the praying motion to convince parties of his neutrality and honest broker status. The second useful gesture is the shoulder shrug. A shrug of both shoulders generally indicates that the person is not interested in the item currently under discussion. A single shoulder movement indicates a desire to be left out. Here the conciliator's main interest will be observing shoulder shrugs by the parties, and using the

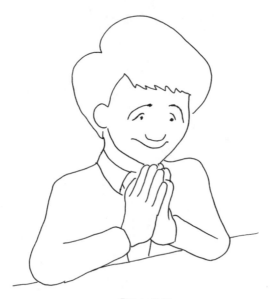

Figure 9.15

signal as a trigger to change the subject, using the 'don't care' aspect if appropriate (Figure 9.16).

Another gesture is the touching of various parts of the body. Many people will touch their chin or pull their ear just after they have got away with something. A car driver, for example, often pulls his ear after a near escape. In the conciliation setting, a person who displays this gesture may feel that they have just achieved an unlikely success. The conciliator may want to look back over the previous two minutes to discover what they think they have 'got away with'.

The last area of body language to be considered is touching. In some areas of work, such as counselling, various forms of touching are an important part of body language. For the conciliator, touching is less important. The main touching habit to be considered is the handshake. In the UK, business handshakes between male and female are a comparatively new phenomenon, and many people are slightly embarrassed by the action. The end result is that when shaking hands with a person of the opposite sex, the male tends to give a limp, weak hold, whilst the female can be over-aggressive in the handshake. The conciliator needs to develop a firm but not over-strong style for use with all parties. He also needs to watch carefully as the parties shake hands on arrival, to detect any early attempt at dominance through a strong grip. Cultural differences occur even within Europe on the handshake question. Most other countries within Europe are more used to the two sexes shaking hands. Some countries add an embrace or light kiss between sexes, even some same-sex handshakes are accompanied by an embrace on second or subsequent meetings. The British tend to hold back more than other Europeans on most aspects of touching.

Some people, nonetheless, are quite tactile. They will touch their nearest neighbour on the knee, the hand, the shoulder. Some persons, when touched, will shrug the touch off. Such behaviour may happen within the conciliation scenario. The rejection of the touch provides better clues for the conciliator than the touch itself. A touch may or may not mean that

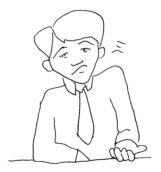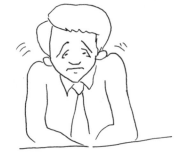

Figure 9.16

there is a feeling of liking the other. Accepting the touch, however, clearly indicates warmth or respect, whilst shrugging off shows dislike. Both are useful relationship clues for the conciliator.

The conciliator will need to observe the body language of the parties in all situations. This is comparatively straightforward when in a separate meeting with just one person. In a complex joint meeting, with several parties, and each party represented by several people, the observation becomes more difficult. The conciliator will need to watch not only the reaction of the persons in the party to persons in other parties, but also the interaction of the people within a party group. The party group will attempt to have a confidential chat between themselves. Indeed, the conciliator may need to ensure that the room layout allows this to occur. When discussing a point within a party team, the group members' body language may signify a response to the proposal currently 'on the table', or it may signify a response to a point made by another member of the same team during the confidential chat. As a general rule, if the party group are discussing a point made by a member of another party group, they will glance at the person who made the suggestion from time to time. If they are discussing a point made entirely by themselves, they will tend to reserve their eye contact for each other. This is not an absolute rule, and the conciliator will need to note other aspects of body language to identify whether a nod of the head indicates acceptance of the other party's point, or agreement with his own team member that they should do something, possibly even reject the other party's suggestion. Clues will come from the way the members of the team react to each other. A high level of reflecting, moving closer together, touching each other accompanied by surreptitiously looking at the other party and avoiding eye contact, would suggest that the group are uniting against the other party. A higher degree of body movement, turning the whole body towards the other party, making occasional eye contact with the other party might indicate that they are deciding to accept the point made by that party.

It is worth mentioning that body language is affected by distance and proximity. Out of doors, and at greater distances, we tend to exaggerate our body language. Indoors, or when very close to other people, we tend to minimize the movements. This is a subconscious change, and means that the conciliator may need to watch for body language signals more intensely during the 'coffee chat' stage if people are close together when talking.

Body language is a vast subject. It has been the intention of this brief description to provide some basic, pragmatic guidance for the conciliator. The conciliator who wishes to know more is advised to read one of the more specialized books, or to attend a practical training programme on the subject.

10

Benefits and shortfalls of conciliation

Conciliation is comparatively reactive, mediation is more pro-active. The use of conciliation in resolving NHS complaints is bound to become more widespread as time passes. The mere fact that the process is being widely used in family law, retail trades, holiday industry and a wide variety of other commercial and industrial situations means that its use will spread. Conciliation is not, however, a panacea for all the problems of the NHS relationship with its patients. By the time conciliation is used in resolving a complaint, or mediation comes into a medical dispute, it is probably too late for good relationships to be set up (Case Study 10).

Case Study 10

An American doctor was visiting the UK recently, and had the misfortune to suffer two minor accidents which required hospital treatment. After visiting two NHS hospitals, his verdict was that 'Your hospitals are not patient friendly'. He was asked to explain the statement. He said that in both hospitals he recognized that the treatment he was receiving (first for a broken wrist, latterly for a broken thumb), was correct, professional and well applied. The communication he received, however, was minimal. Nobody told him what was happening or explained the treatment, timescales, end effects etc. In both cases in due time he let it be known to the staff that he was a doctor. In both hospitals, as soon as they discovered he was a doctor the handling of his case changed. There was no treatment change, but the treatment was explained, clarified, discussed. The staff exchanged chat and confidences. The American doctor was quite convinced that an ordinary patient would have left with overall negative feelings. Indeed, he stated that the only reason he did not complain about staff attitudes was that he was not asked to pay for his treatment. A conciliatory approach to this patient from the start, instead of part way through his treatment on discovering his profession, would have meant a much happier patient. This case may evoke a reaction from those who feel that American standards are not relevant to today's

Case Study 10: *continued*

NHS in the UK. It may also suggest that the conciliatory approach is nothing new. In the past it may have been there, but simply called a good bedside manner. In either event, it is suggested that to communicate openly, fully and effectively with patients at all stages of contact can only be a good thing.

Conciliation can only work if all the parties concerned have a degree of willingness to achieve a positive result. If there is one unwilling party, conciliation is unlikely to succeed. The situations in which conciliation is unlikely to succeed were briefly discussed in Chapter 3 and are dealt with fully in Chapter 10. Where conciliation is well applied, it can achieve results in settling disputes which have seemed intractable. The introduction of a good, well trained and experienced conciliator as an honest broker can break down barriers and bring about open and frank discussion. In most circumstances, the settlement of a dispute can only come from discussion.

One prime benefit from good conciliation is that it can avoid litigation. Where a dispute exists between a complainant and an NHS provider, resorting to litigation is not likely to settle a dispute but merely make it go away. If the complainant should lose the case, he will continue to feel aggrieved at the action of the NHS provider. If the complainant wins, the trust or primary provider professional will often harbour on-going ill will towards the patient or the legal system. Even the patient who has won his case, and possibly been awarded substantial monies, may still not be satisfied with the outcome, particularly if the outcome he wanted was an acceptance of blame or liability. The provider may simply pay the money and continue to deny responsibility.

Conciliation, on the other hand, results in agreement between the parties. Even if one aspect of the dispute is left on a basis of 'agree to disagree', that feeling of achievement for both parties remains. Thus conciliation can achieve genuine satisfaction for both parties. As an alternative to litigation, conciliation is more cost effective and will often produce a more acceptable result. It is even possible during the conciliation process to handle the question of compensation, if the complainant is justly entitled to some recompense to reduce the negative effects of the problem. To reach agreement on compensation in this process is more cost effective than resorting to litigation. It would, of course, be wise to seek relevant professional advice on amounts and confirmations of such agreements. Where there is a possibility of the matter of compensation arising, it is also wise for the conciliator to ensure that the complained against have the necessary authority. This may involve discussion with, or inclusion of, representatives of the insurers, such as the Medical Defence Union.

Conciliation is cost effective. The total time taken by the conciliator to resolve a case will be measured in hours rather than days or weeks. Many full conciliations, conducted within a single building, in their entirety, will take minutes rather than hours. As many conciliators will be existing employees using only a small part of their time, and others will be volunteers, the cost of the conciliator's time can be quite low. It is inevitable that commercial conciliation will be used. Even in the first few months of the new complaints procedures, commercial conciliation was offered to NHS providers in South East England. The use of a professional conciliator will clearly add to the cost, but if such conciliators are efficient and well trained, they may be more cost effective than resorting to the high costs of using external lawyers.

In recent times, some patients or carers have decided to involve the media when they were dissatisfied with the handling of a complaint. The adverse effects of media publicity on a trust or primary provider cannot be overstated. Noticeable among the comments given a high profile in such stories is that it is often the handling of the complaint, as much as the original issue, which is highlighted. Very often the published interview will contain phrases such as 'in the three months after my wife's death, nobody from the trust even contacted me!' Another very common comment is 'they may have admitted liability, but nobody from that practice has ever said sorry. All I want is for someone to just say sorry!' By its very nature, a conciliatory approach should prevent a fair number of such stories ever being given to the press. One piece of adverse publicity avoided through the application of good handling of the complaint, including the conciliatory approach and even formal conciliation, will justify all the effort in developing a conciliation service.

Time and resources are often quoted as being in short supply throughout the NHS. A good complaints handling procedure, including conciliation, can achieve the Wilson Report's aim of resolving the majority of complaints locally and quickly. The time saved for health professionals and NHS managers will again more than justify the introduction of a conciliatory approach.

Failure to resolve a complaint locally will bring in the activities of outside persons. For the primary sector it will be the Health Authority or Health Board, in the form of the convenor and independent review panel. Non-executive directors acting as convenors, followed by lay persons nominated by the NHS Executive Region, or the Health Board, will become involved in trust complaints. On top of these, the Ombudsman lurks ready to pounce. Successful local resolution will prevent all of this. A good conciliation and conciliatory approach can prove their worth once more.

Conciliation is not, however, a process to be used exclusively with fully trained and external conciliators. Most of the NHS trusts that have decided to use conciliation have, in fact, selected and trained a group of existing employees or managers to act as conciliators, or to apply a conciliatory approach to the early handling of complaints. The real benefits of conciliation are probably seen more effectively where the nurse, receptionist, junior doctor or other person who is the first contact with the complainant adopts the conciliatory approach quite naturally. This application of conciliation is clearly illustrated in the following case (Case Study 11), which is told in the words of the receptionist concerned.

Case Study 11

It was 8.30 a.m. one Monday morning, and the first patient I dealt with was a very tearful university student accompanied by her mother. She said that she wanted to speak to somebody regarding a complaint against one of our GPs. As she was so upset I took her to the practice manager's room (the practice manger was on holiday at the time). I calmed her and then asked her to explain the problem to me. She stated that she had recently sat a very important exam and had received a very poor grade. She had spoken to her tutors explaining that the reason for the poor result was that she was under a lot of personal strain. They replied that if she wanted to re-sit the exam she would need a letter from her GP confirming these facts. She obtained a letter from one of our GPs but her re-sit application was refused. She told me that she was very unhappy with the contents of the letter as she felt that the GP had not explained her problems fully. The details were that her father was very ill, the family business was failing, and she and her mother were tending to her father, the business, and trying to protect the younger members of the family from the problems. On top of this she had the added worry of the exam. I took all of the details down and listened in a sympathetic manner. I asked her if I could go and speak to the GP in question, and she agreed. When I spoke to him about the problem, I found that he knew nothing of the family problems. Another GP in the practice had been attending her father, and she had not explained her problems fully. He agreed to see her again to discuss matters further if she wished to do so. I explained this to the patient and she agreed that she had not given the doctor the full details of her problems as she assumed he would have known about her father. After I explained that not all patients' cases are discussed between all of the partners, and that when a patient consulted a GP they should give all the details of any problem to him otherwise a proper diagnosis could not be made, she thanked me for the explanation and said she would like to see the GP again. She did so the same morning and was much happier when she left the practice.

This case illustrates many aspects of successful conciliation. All of the steps of conciliation are identifiable. The conciliator acted as an honest broker. Movement occurred before the parties came together. Agreement and satisfaction were the end result. And yet the receptionist concerned had not been to full and detailed training on conciliation skills. She had attended the Advanced Receptionist Development Programme, but this includes only a small element of definition of conciliation. The receptionist had applied good customer care, common sense and first class communication techniques. The end result was that a conciliatory approach, without formal conciliation, resolved a situation happily. The incident will probably not even achieve the status of a statistic in the practice complaint records. This case shows a very clear illustration of the benefits of conciliation in dealing with dissatisfied patients.

When it works well, conciliation has many advantages, and few disadvantages. The shortfalls of conciliation come in the main from situations where it does not, or cannot, work well. The first cause of failure has to be the shortage of trained and experienced conciliators (Case Study 12).

Case Study 12

In one Health Authority area their very experienced conciliator, a man with extensive experience of arbitration and mediation, was asked to recruit and train a group of lay persons as conciliators. He recruited from among the Health Authority list of volunteers, and had about 50 willing candidates. He reduced the number to 20 by interview and discussion, and commenced a training programme with the 20 people. Three months after the training ended, two of the original group were actually involved in conciliation. Eighteen had either decided that conciliation was not for them, or the Health Authority had decided that they were, even after training, not suitable to become conciliators. Another Health Authority decided to appoint 16 former service committee members as conciliators. After a very short period it was discovered that the reputation of the service committee members as combative, adversarial participants in the former discipline procedure meant that they were all rejected by the providers. The Health Authority has now implemented a training programme for new volunteer lay conciliators.

Before conciliation is attempted, it is essential to have confidence that it will succeed. An attempt to conciliate which fails is quite likely to leave the situation worse than before. Consider the situation in which both parties, the complainant and the complained against, have fully participated in all the local resolution attempts to deal with the problem. The complainant will have been seen (interrogated?) by their first contact, a junior professional, a manager, a doctor and a complaints manager, which amounts to five interviews. If the complaint is complex, involving, say, a primary provider, an ambulance trust, a community health trust and a social services department, the complainant may have been 'interrogated' 10 or 20 times. Then, as a last resort, along comes the conciliator like a knight in shining armour. From the point of view of the parties, this is just one more push towards their already entrenched positions. The late attempt at conciliation has a high probability of failure. The end result will be that the parties are further apart than ever. Both managers of complaints and conciliators must be able to recognize a lost cause and not commence further activity. The preventative measure in a case such as this is to involve one conciliator to act across all parties at a very early stage (Case Study 13).

Case Study 13

A teenage girl saw her GP is early September. The GP suspected an eating disorder and referred the patient as a routine, non-urgent case to the local community and mental health trust. No further contact occurred between the GP and the patient. The patient's father contacted the trust several times by telephone to ask when his daughter would be seen, but received no response. In early January, the patient was rushed into a private eating disorder hospital unit in a very serious condition. The father visited the Community Health Council (CHC) to complain. The CHC manager was very disturbed at the story he heard and contacted the patient service manager of the trust immediately. The patient service manager had no prior knowledge of the situation. He received the notification at 8.30 a.m. and immediately carried out such checks as he could, and discovered that the original referral letter had been mis-filed. The telephone calls from the father had been ignored deliberately as the consultant felt that professionally he could not deal with the family of a patient who had not been properly referred. The GP was unaware that the patient had deteriorated, and had made no attempt to follow up in any way. The patient services manager invited all the parties to a meeting at 11.00 a.m. and all parties, except the consultant surgeon, attended. Within 20 minutes the trust had apologised for its error in filing, and offered to set up a new procedure to prevent a recurrence. The GP had apologised for not following up, and offered to set up a parallel procedure. The trust promised to set up an investigation into the lack

Case Study 13: *continued*

of response to the father's telephone calls. Even the father apologised for not pushing hard enough on behalf of his daughter. The patient was moved into the care of the trust immediately, and all parties were satisfied. Approximately one hour's work by one person, and a short meeting of eight persons, completely resolved the immediate problem. Plans were set in motion to prevent recurrence. All of this was achieved because the patient services manager adopted a conciliatory style from the start.

The biggest disadvantage of conciliation is probably that it is not binding on the parties. It is, therefore, a requirement of the conciliator's technique that he gains a very strong commitment to the agreement by the parties. This cannot be done if the parties involved in the conciliation process do not have the authority to reach and abide by the agreement. In most cases, the patient will, of course, be present and have the authority. In primary sector cases, the practitioner will normally also be present and have authority. The problem can arise, however, where a purchaser decision is the issue at stake. The only person relevant as a party at the conciliation meeting is the person with authority to vary the purchasing decision. If the decision is deemed absolutely irreversible, then concilia-tion should not be attempted. The lack of authority may also be an issue where the complainant will only be satisfied with an apology. Whether or not an apology is appropriate, only the person with authority to agree, or deny, such an apology can represent the party. This can easily arise where the apology has to come from a clinical or medical professional. It is no good the trust quality assurance director promising an apology if the consultant surgeon later refuses to apologise. Whether or not he should apologise is irrelevant. If an apology from the consultant is a potential outcome of conciliation, then the consultant must participate willingly in the process of conciliation.

It has been stated earlier that the time to be allocated for conciliation is open ended, but normally comparatively short. It is, even so, a disadvantage that the time is difficult to estimate accurately. In some cases, where there is a very wide range of issues to be resolved, or very entrenched positions have already been adopted, it is possible that conciliation could require a considerable time commitment. Normally, the majority of such time will be for the conciliator to spend with each party separately. Thus, although the commitment of the conciliator himself may be extensive, the time spent by professionals and other employees is minimized. The actual joint meeting, even in a complex case, should be a few hours at the very most, normally less. The conciliator should not embark on an attempt at conciliation if the time commitment can be foreseen as greater than any of the parties can or will commit.

There are some situations which require special attention. One of the most common areas within the NHS which receives complaints is the mental health sector. Patients who are mentally ill may not want to be treated or detained in a forensic unit. Mentally ill patients sometimes suffer delusions as a part of their illness. The most common delusions are poisoning by doctors or staff, theft of or damage to property, and physical or sexual assault. The conciliator who becomes involved in resolving a case with a mentally ill patient must be aware of the implications of delusions on the conciliation process. The first, and obvious, effect is that a complainant who is mentally ill may be bringing a complaint which is entirely without justification, but to the patient it is very real. The second danger is that where the complaint is genuine, based on actual events, the people handling the complaint may dismiss it as a delusion. All the persons involved with a mentally ill complainant must be aware of the complications. They must also be clever enough to spot the 'real' problem, particularly where a patient has a history of proven or accepted delusions. Where a patient is detained in a forensic unit against his will, particularly long term, he will sometimes make a complaint as a means of attracting attention or giving himself an interesting diversion from the dull routine of the day. In some cases he will make a complaint as a malicious way of causing problems for the unit staff. On being committed to a forensic unit by a court some patients consider themselves to be prisoners, and even refer to the staff as 'screws'. Such patients will also have access to first class help from counsellors and others in forming and presenting their complaints. Clearly the dangers for the conciliator with little or no experience of working with the mentally ill can be quite extensive and varied. The consequences of failure by the conciliator, and indeed all of those working with complaints in this sector, can be quite severe. The antidote is for the conciliator to seek the advice of an uninvolved psychiatric expert as part of his preparation to conciliate in such a case.

Another common situation which needs special attention is a complaint concerning a bereavement. Bereaved families pass through a number of stages in the bereavement process. Some of these stages of bereavement can lead to the family making and pressing a complaint which is more a part of their own handling of their loss than an actual grievance. One of the stages which occurs is guilt. This is particularly likely to happen where the family is geographically dispersed, or where the patient has died of a hereditary condition. The latter is particularly strong where the deceased is a young child. The conciliator is advised to familiarize himself with the stages of bereavement and their effects as part of the preparation for conciliation where a death has occurred and is part of the base of the complaint. This does not mean that every time the conciliator comes across a case revolving around a death, that he is dealing with a nonproblem. The complainant will undoubtedly feel very strongly that he has genuine reason for dissatisfaction. But in some cases he may be, in fact, trying to transfer his guilt. A very good way for the conciliator to make himself aware of the matters concerning bereavement, without the need to become an expert bereavement counsellor, is to obtain and read a selection of the excellent leaflets produced by CRUSE, the bereavement counselling charity which has local offices throughout the UK.

11

When conciliation may not work

Conciliation is a very powerful technique which can be relied upon, when well implemented, to resolve a wide range of problems. Even so, there are some situations in which even conciliation cannot be expected to succeed. In previous chapters it has been established that conciliation may not achieve a lasting result where the parties do not have authority, where one or more parties is inclined to violence or to serious neurotic behaviour, or where the parties have difficulty in communicating. This chapter looks at situations where conciliation is extremely unlikely to achieve any result at all, let alone a result which may be later set aside by one of the parties.

The first serious barrier to conciliation arises where one or other of the parties refuses to co-operate. It is unlikely that a complainant will refuse if conciliation is introduced properly, at an early stage, but it is possible that the party complained against will decline to join. Where conciliation is introduced late, particularly where a review panel request has been sent back for conciliation by the convenor, the complainant is very likely to refuse to participate. The conciliator's role and conciliatory style do mean that he can try to persuade the parties to take part. If the parties cannot be convinced, then conciliation simply cannot commence. The conciliator should record on the file that one or both parties did not agree to take part, and that conciliation is not possible.

Another situation in which the conciliator may have to decide that conciliation is not possible is a case in which his early analysis identifies that the two parties are widely split on attitudes. If all the facts are agreed, if there are no opinions involved, but the parties have widely differing and deeply held attitudes, there is no point to attempting to roll the conciliation process beyond the initial meetings and analysis. Attitudes, by definition, cannot be moved by discussion or persuasion. Where those attitudes are tending towards the extreme depth of prejudice, there is absolutely no chance of conciliation working. This situation poses greater difficulties for the conciliator. Here, the reason for not proceeding is a decision based on the opinion of the conciliator. It will be necessary to double check that the classification of the entrenched views as 'attitude' is absolutely correct. Probably it will be wise for the conciliator to check with a third party, preferably another experienced conciliator. If the decision is taken not to proceed, the file should again have a note appended to the effect that in the conciliator's opinion the division between the parties is too great for conciliation to succeed. It would not be helpful for the conciliator to actually specify 'attitude' or 'prejudice'. It will then be up to managers to decide on further action.

Even more contentious is the case of the chronic complainant. The chronic complainant is a person who frequently, and without necessarily having acceptable grounds, complains. Fortunately there are very few chronic complainants in the UK. Chronic complainants will often be known to the local health authority, since they will have a history of frequent complaints against a variety of providers. It must be noted that a person who make series of complaints against the same provider is not necessarily a chronic complainant. Such people are often forced into a series of complaints due a lack of satisfaction at each stage, and so they push harder and longer to obtain a satisfactory response. Chronic complainants can be classified as people who make it very clear that whatever happens, they will take it all the way. Experienced managers of complaints will spot a chronic complainant within the first few minutes. The first clues to identify a chronic complainant will usually come from the managers of the complaints. Words such 'nothing will satisfy this one', 'he has already said he is going to the Secretary of State' will have been used regularly. The conciliator will, however, have to make his own judgement. If the conciliator decides in such a case that conciliation will not work, he must still decide whether or not to try. The format of the NHS procedure is such that it may be necessary to attempt conciliation even in such a case. If conciliation is not attempted, then the chronic complainant will have one more potential piece of ammunition to use. In such a case the decision should be made in conjunction with the managers of the complaint, and recorded on the file accordingly.

Finally, it may be that the conciliator himself is rejected by one of the parties. This does not mean that conciliation cannot be attempted. It merely means that an alternative conciliator may need to be offered. The grounds for rejection of a conciliator will vary, and mean that health authorities and trusts may need to have available not only a number of conciliators, but also a number of sources of conciliators. Some possible grounds for rejection may be:

- Bias – One or other of the parties may believe that as the conciliator is directly associated wth the practice, trust or authority involved in the complaint, then the conciliator is bound to be biased. This is most likely to be a feeling by the complainant, but may also occur where, for example, trust staff feel that the conciliator is part of management, and management are biased against staff.
- Personality – The party may simply not like the conciliator on first impression. This could occur in almost any circumstance, even by telephone. The conciliator should be on guard and be aware that the first impression created is extremely important, and should always be positive.

- Race, creed or religion – Prejudice exists in all quarters of a multi-racial society. Prejudice does not carry any degree of logic, and rejection on these grounds may be insuperable. The availability of conciliators from a variety of ethnic backgrounds will be a help, but it is quite likely that if one party rejects a conciliator on grounds of race, the other party may reject the second choice conciliator.

12

Communicating with the parties to the conciliation process

Communicating with the parties is at all times subject to all the rules and problems of human communication. One point is quite probable, namely that if the parties have reached a point at which they cannot resolve their own differences, there will almost certainly be existing communication problems between them. In some cases the original issue will in itself have been a communication problem. In other cases communications may have broken down as a result of failed attempts to resolve the dispute.

In communication with the parties, the 'I' factor and the 'eye' factor must be taken into account. The 'I' factor is simply that for the vast majority of human beings, the most important person in the world is himself. We are all basically selfish to some degree. Thus, any communication from any source is most likely to be accepted if it appeals to the 'I' factor. A simple example of the 'I' factor at work could be the agreement of timing for a meeting. If the conciliator wants to agree 3.00 p.m., he might say 'I will be in your area at about 3.00 p.m., and it will help me if you can see me then'. This will offer no personal benefit to the party, who may or may not accept. Alternatively, if the conciliator says 'I know you have to collect the children at 4.00 p.m., so why don't I come at 3.00 p.m?', success is almost assured. The same timing, but consideration for the 'I' factor of the party.

This respect for the 'I' factor may extend to all parts of the conciliation process. If the conciliator can spot 'I' factor clues as the parties discuss the issues, and in an ideal situation offer personal benefits alternately to each party, then he will be able bring the parties forward relatively well to an agreed conclusion. Likewise, in the pre-meetings if he can spot and amplify 'I' factor benefits as the party begins to move on facts and opinions, progress could be rapid.

The 'I' factor also applies, of course, to the final confirmation of agreement. Whether the written confirmation is prepared on the spot, or sent later by the conciliator, 'I' factor benefits can be highlighted. This may be slightly easier to achieve where the confirmation is sent after the event, as this will enable the conciliator to compose two similar, but subtly different, letters. If any single factor of human communication is of prime importance to the conciliator, it is this use of the 'I' factor.

The 'eye' factor is the maximization of the use of the sense of sight, and the elimination of the distraction of the eyes, which has already been discussed in an earlier paragraph. The sense of sight can be utilized fairly well in the meetings. In the pre-meetings, the conciliator and the party can compose the list of agreed points together, the conciliator writing on a pad with the party watching and agreeing each point. In the joint meeting, the conciliator may, from time to time, again use a piece of paper to summarize, thus focusing the attention of both parties. This paper summary is occasionally a useful device when things get a little fraught. The action of the conciliator saying 'let me just make a note of these points, they are very important to you both ...' can be quite a calming influence if used sparingly. The importance of the eyes in listening and body language has already been extensively discussed, and is an important part of the 'eye' factor.

Apart from the two 'I's, it is very important to emphasize the positive and minimize the negative throughout conciliation. Human beings always react negatively to a negative start. Many react positively to a positive trigger. A probability of the positive is far superior to a guarantee of the negative. The conciliator will need to practice the art of finding good news at the heart of every point: not only finding it, but high-lighting it and having it accepted by the parties.

Reflection as a listening technique has been mentioned. It can, however, be extended beyond the simple confirmation of points and opinions made by the parties. Reflecting the style and content of the parties' own communications can be helpful. This does not mean that the conciliator has to repeat any foul language used by the party, but the style and type of vocabulary are important. Different researchers vary in their estimates of the number of words used by people. It is likely that most of us survive on a vocabulary of a few hundred words a day. Some believe that women use a wider vocabulary than men. People who read the broadsheet newspapers certainly use a wider vocabulary than tabloid readers. The conciliator needs to be sensitive to the extent of vocabulary used by the party, and respond in a similar vein. Reflection may also apply to the format of communication. If it is clear that one of the parties prefers to communicate by letter, then the conciliator may have to start with a letter, probably one inviting the party to a discussion.

Jargon is also a problem in some cases. There was one complaint recently where a patient stated that he had not been told that he had cancer. The doctor was quite specific, he had informed the patient that he had a tumour. Most of us would associate the word tumour with cancer. This patient did not. The communication failure was on the part of the doctor: he should have checked understanding. The conciliator may have to be a 'jargon' decipherer for the complainant. This point may be particularly important for mediators resolving differences over treatment. All professional people are inclined to use technical language. Often detailed technical language is essential to enable the medics to know exactly what they are discussing. 'MCI' , for example, means 'Management Charter Initiative' to people in the education world. To a doctor, MCI is a specific type of heart attack, Myo Cardial Infarction. The mediator, and sometimes the conciliator, should train himself to spot such jargon, and ask the user to explain it in lay language. Dentists, opticians, pharmacists and nurses all have their own vocabulary, which is a mystery to the lay person. All complainants can be treated as lay persons.

Appendix 1 – Flow chart of the conciliation process

THE CONCILIATION PROCESS

Party A tell conciliator their 'story'

Party B tell conciliator their 'story'

Conciliator summarizes party A story to party A

Conciliator summarizes party B story to party B

Conciliator privately analyses both stories
identifies common ground
identifies disagreement

Conciliator divides items into
facts, opinions and attitudes

Conciliator checks disputed facts
to identify genuine facts

Conciliator identifies further
common ground

Conciliator summarizes Party A common ground to party A

Conciliator summarizes Party B common ground to party B

Conciliator summarizes Party B common ground to party A

Conciliator summarizes Party A common ground to party B

Conciliator gains agreement of both parties
to each other's common ground

Conciliator introduces disputed facts
to both parties, introduces his factual checks,
gains agreement of both parties to actual facts

Conciliator has now reduced the disagreement to opinions
and attitudes. The real conciliation is about to commence.
In a 'normal' situation, the disagreement now concerns a
small number of strongly felt issues.

Conciliator separates opinions from attitudes

Conciliator discusses opinions of party B with party A	Conciliator discusses opinions of party A with party B
Conciliator discusses responses of party B with party A	Conciliator discusses responses of party A with party B

Conciliator gains agreement from each party
that other party has a basis for opinions

Conciliator brings parties together to discuss
differing opinions under his/her chairmanship

Parties opinions move closer together, agreement
reached point by point until substantial agreement

Conciliator introduces attitudes (without using word
'attitude') to achieve agreement of right to hold thoughts

Conciliator summarizes issues, highlighting high volume
agreement and low level difference

Conciliator leads parties to agreement that differences will
not be resolved, but will be left and mutually acknowledged

Conciliator confirms in writing to both parties immediately

KEY: ☐ = Conciliator alone with party A;   ⬭ = Conciliator alone with
party B;   ▧ = Conciliator alone;   ■ = Conciliator with both parties.

Appendix 2 – Check list for the conciliator

	Yes	No

- Have you received the contact points for all the parties?
- Can you start discussion with a clear mind?
- Do you need any additional information?
- Do you know or suspect what the true problem is?
- Do the parties concerned know or suspect what the true problem is?
- If not, will they recognize the real problem?
- Have they indicated any wish for conciliation or help?
- If the previous two responses were 'NO', do you have unwilling parties?
- Can you allow enough time to do the conciliation properly?
- Can they allow enough time?
- Can you find a quiet place without interruptions?
- Will they accept your promise of 'neutrality'?
- Is there an existing base of trust between you?
- Do you know enough about the parties involved?
- Are you on your guard against taking sides?
- Is each side willing to move from its starting position?
- What is the ideal settlement each party would like to achieve?
- What is the minimum settlement each party is likely to accept?
- Are you prepared to allow both parties to talk? And to listen?
- Are you prepared to observe body language?
- How will you avoid or prevent such phrases as 'My fair and reasonable position'?
- Can you identify stages of agreement to be aimed at?
- Have you identified facts?

Appendix 2: *continued*   *Yes   No*

- Have you identified opinions?
- Have you isolated attitudes?
- Can you illustrate points of agreement?
- Can you isolate attitudes?
- Are you prepared to explain WHY certain items are facts?
- Are you prepared to summarize viewpoints, emphasizing points of agreement, at all stages?
- Are you ready to spot and highlight conciliatory gestures?
- What is the complainant's expected level of response?
- Has that expectation been recognized, acknowledged or met?
- Can that expectation be reasonably met?
- Will (or should) that expectation be acceptable to the complained against?
- Can that expectation be met so that both parties can claim they have gained something of value?
- Can that expectation be met so that neither party loses face?
- Has communication to date been good from and to both parties?
- Has time lapse caused the complaint to grow or change from its original form?
- How will you follow it up?

Glossary

ACAS	The Advisory, Conciliation and Arbitration Service set up by the UK Government to assist in the resolution of disputes between employers and employees.
Apology	A sincere expression of regret.
Arbitration	The process of settling a disagreement between two or more parties by the introduction of an external body or person with authority to make and implement an agreement.
Attitude	A view or opinion which is so strongly held that it cannot be altered by normal, reasonable argument or proof.
Body language	Non-verbal communication, mainly subconscious, whereby messages are sent and received between people through the stance or movement of all or part of the body.
Chairman	A person who leads or conducts discussions. A chairman's skill and technique may be used in a one-to-one meeting, or by indirect communication methods such as the telephone.
CHC	Community Health Council – local bodies set up to protect the interests of NHS users.
Comment	An expression of opinion which falls short of a formal suggestion or complaint.
Communication	The two-way process of exchanging ideas, thought, feelings and facts.
Complaint	An expression of dissatisfaction.
Complainant	The person who expresses the dissatisfaction. They may or may not be the patient concerned.
Compliment	An expression of approval or satisfaction.
Conciliation	The process of a lay person assisting two parties in dispute to reach informal agreement through discussion and persuasion, without any legally binding status.
Conciliatory approach	The application of conciliation techniques outside a formal conciliation process.
Convenor	A non-executive director of a trust, health authority or health board who decides whether or not to

	convene an independent panel to review a complaint against an NHS provider.
Customer	A person who uses a service.
Designated person	A person within an NHS provider, or a department of an NHS provider, who is delegated responsibility to ensure that complaints are properly resolved locally.
Emotion	An intense feeling which may not have a rational foundation.
Fact	Something that exists or occurs and can be proven by objective evidence.
FHS	Family Health Services – the primary health care providers, including GPs, dentists, pharmacists, opticians.
Front line staff	The employees of an NHS provider who have direct face-to-face contact with patients and other NHS users.
Health Service Commissioner	The Ombudsman, appointed by Parliament to protect the rights of users of the NHS. Responsible only to Parliament.
Hearing	The process of perceiving sound.
Independent review	The process of a panel of lay persons reviewing the case of a complaint where the complainant is not satisfied with the results of local resolution by an NHS provider.
Inspiration trap	The difficulty faced by a conciliator who can identify an obvious and sensible solution to a dispute, but must ensure that the parties to the dispute reach the same conclusion without identifiable direction from the conciliator.
Lay	A person who is not, and preferably never has been, a professional in the field under dispute or any associated field.
Listen	The process of actively hearing, accepting and understanding a verbal communication.
Local resolution	The process of resolving a complaint against an NHS provider swiftly, at or very near to the point at which the issue complained about actually occurred.
Logical	To follow a sound set of rules and tests.
Mediation	The process of resolving a dispute by the intervention of an expert person who closely guides the disputing parties towards agreement.
Mind map	A process of recording information in related groupings which is intended to assist lateral thinking.

Movement	The stage in a conciliation or mediation process during which the parties modify their views and their opinions become closer to each other's.
Objective	A clearly identifiable and quantifiable target to be achieved in the future.
Opinion	A belief which is held but may not be based on provable fact.
Patient	A person currently or previously under medical care.
Party	A patient, carer, representative or NHS provider involved in a dispute.
Personality	The distinctive and identifiable characteristics of an individual human being.
Prejudice	An opinion for or against something without logical basis and held so strongly that it cannot be modified in any way except to be strengthened.
Procedure	A particular and specified way of doing something.
Protocol	An alternative word for procedure.
Quality	A specified standard of performance.
Quango	A Quasi-Autonomous Non-Governmental Organization. A body with virtual statutory power.
Reflection	The process of returning verbal or body language communication to the original perpetrator to indicate agreement and acceptance.
Relate	A voluntary body, formerly known as the Marriage Guidance Council, which assists couples to resolve differences which threaten their relationship.
Rudyard Kipling's Serving Men	'I keep six honest serving men (They taught me all I know): Their names are What and Why and When and How and Where and Who.'
Seeding	The process of 'planting' all or part of an idea or plan in the mind(s) of others such that those persons produce the plan as if it were their own original thought.
Suggestion	The process of putting a thought, plan or desire to another person.
Training	The process of modifying behaviour at work through instruction, example or practice.
Tribunal	A court-like procedure for the resolution of disputes.
Wilson Report	A report titled 'Being Heard', the report of a review committee on NHS complaints procedures published in May 1994.

Further reading

Bone D A (1988) *A Practical Guide to Effective Listening*. London: Kogan Page.

Buzan T (1995) *The Mind Map Book*. London: BBC Books.

Ford J K and Merriman P (1990) *The Gentle Art of Listening*. London: Bedford Square Press.

Lyle J (1991) *Body Language*. London: Hamlyn.

MOR (1995) *Complaints Handling in the Public Sector*. London: HMSO.

Morris D (1994) *The Naked Ape Trilogy*. London: Cape.

Pease A (1992) *Body Language*. London: Sheldon Press.

Pickersgill D and Stanton A (eds) (1997) *Making Sense of the NHS Complaints and Disciplinary Procedures*. Oxford: Radcliffe Medical Press.

Stuttard M (1988) *Body Language*. Shortland Publications.

Wainwright G R (1985) *Body Language*. London: Hodder & Stoughton.

Index

ACAS (Arbitration, Conciliation and
    Advisory Service) 2
  equivalent in Australia 3
'Acting on complaints' 5
addiction, see mental illness
Advanced Receptionist Development
    Programme 69
  see also staff, training of
'agreed disagreement' 27
agreement
  maintaining 13, 71
  reaching 13
aggression 46, see also violence
ambulance trust 12–13
apology, appropriateness of 71
arbitration 36
  definition of 1, 2
  see also 'Pendulum arbitration'
attitudes 33, 47, 74, 76
  definition of 26
  overcoming 34
Australia, equivalent of ACAS in, see ACAS

'Being Heard', see Wilson Report
beliefs 14
  see also opinions
bereavement 72
  preparation for conciliator in dealing
    with 72–3
  see also CRUSE (bereavement counselling
    charity)
bias 15, 75
'blank mind', see impartiality
blood transfusion 20
body language 3, 24, 30, 32, 34, 51–64
  and conciliator's role 52
  cultural differences 51–2
  eyes 54–6
    eye contact 3, 24, 43, 54–6
    glancing technique 43

'staring out' 54, 56
    eyebrows 53
    facial expression 51, 52, 53, 54
    frown 53
    fully open position 61
    gestures 51, 62–3
    head 53, 57–9
    posture 51, 56, 57, 60–2
    shoulders 30, 63
    touching others, see physical contact
    touching parts of own body 63
    when more than two parties
      involved 64
bureaucracy 5, 9

'chat' 18–19, 32, 37, 64
  body language during 64
  in mediation 18
class 47
CHC (Community Health Council) 9
chronic complainants 75
clothing 19, 32, 46
'common ground' 39
communication difficulties 11, 74
communication skills 3, 16
  non-verbal 48, 54
  see also body language
compensation 66
complaints
  investigation of 8
  good managers of 9
  written acknowledgements of 9
complaints handling
  key skills 6
  'on the spot' 8
  single procedure in 5
  see also bureaucracy, Patients' Charter
compliments 6
compromise 2
concentration 46

conciliation
  benefits of 66, 67
  definition of 1, 2
  difficulties in 13
  disadvantages of 71
  limitations of 65–6
  'model' format in 22
  opening of 33
  pre-meetings 33
  steps involved in 39–40, 80–3
  use of within businesses 39
  see also failure in conciliation,
      likelihood of
conciliator
  early use of one for all parties 69
  as 'honest broker' 11, 38, 69
  as lay person 3
  rejection of by party 75, see also race,
      creed and religion
  shortage of 69
  summary of skills required 3
confidentiality in conciliation 16
  legal standing of, see legal system
co-operation, lack of 74
cost 67
cost-effectiveness 67
creed 76
criminal background 47
CRUSE (bereavement counselling
      charity) 73
cultural differences 20
  see also body language, language barriers
customer care 6

deception 14
'designated person' 11
directive approach 39
discussion 29–30
distraction, avoidance of 44
divorce laws 1

eating disorder 68
'egos' of parties 36
emotions 47, 48
employers' responsibility regarding
      mentally ill or violent parties 15
'eye' factor 78
eyes, see under body language, listening
      (tools in)

expectations of parties 36
expertise 12, 17–18

facts 23, 27, 33
  definition of 26
  'holding back of' 28
failure in conciliation, likelihood of 13, 74–5
  see also attitudes, chronic complainants,
      mental illness, violence
feelings, see emotions
food in hospitals 6
front line staff, see staff

glue ear 18–19
'grunting' technique, see mouth

Health Authority 67
health and safety when dealing with
      mentally ill or violent parties 15
Health Board, see Health Authority
Health Service Commissioner, see
      Ombudsman
honesty 14, 19
  use of eyes 55
holiday industry, arbitration in 1
'honest broker', see conciliator
humiliation, see 'egos' of parties

'I' factor 77
impartiality 22, 23, 47
  see also bias, prejudice
'Independent Review' 6, 9, 22
influence 29
informality 31, 32, see also clothing
interpreters, necessary skills 15
investigation 38
  see also complaints

jargon 78
job titles 8

language barriers 15, 20
  see also cultural differences, interpreters,
      jargon
lay persons, see conciliators
legal system (UK)
  relationship to conciliation
      confidentiality 16
  see also divorce laws

lies 14
  eyes as way of detecting 55
listening 12–13, 29
  active techniques in 43–9
  distinction from hearing 42
  in mediation 18
  passive 42
  promotion of listening skills in parties 50
  reasons for 42
  tools in
    body 43, 45, see also body language
    brain 43, 46, 47
    ears 43, 44, 49
    eyes 43–4
    mouth 43, 44
    physical appearance 43, 45
    questioning 46
    time 43
litigation, avoidance of 66
'local resolution' 5, 6, 8, 9, 67
  timing in 8

Marriage Guidance Council, see Relate
media publicity 17, 67
mediation
  definition of 1, 2, 17
  difference from conciliation 17, 20–1, 39
  expert knowledge in 3, 17
  see also listening skills, time
Medical Defence Union 66
Mental Health Act 14
mental health trust 34
mental illness 14, 19, 72, 74
  preparation for conciliator in dealing
      with 14, 72
  see also health and safety, employers'
      responsibility for
'mini agreements' 30
mirroring, see reflection
motivation of staff, see staff
mouth 44
  lip reading 44
  'grunting' technique 45
  see also listening (tools in), voice
'movement' 27, 28, 33, 34, 40
  clues to
    change of direction 35
    change of wording 35
    introductory phrases 35

neurotic behaviour, see mental illness
NHS Executive (NHSE)
  interim guidelines 5
  final guidelines 5
non-directive approach 39
note taking 25, 26, 48–9

objective, importance of establishing 15
Ombudsman (Health Service
      Commissioner) 9, 67
Ombudsman review 6
opinions 33
  definition of 26

parties, separation of 41
Patients' Charter 9
'Pendulum arbitration' 2
personality 3–4, 16, 75
persuasion 18, 19, 29
physical appearance
  height 46
  significance of 45
  see also clothing tools in listening
physical contact 63
politics 17
practice manager complained against 13
prejudice 12
  see also bias, creed, race, religion
protocols (practice or trust) 7
purchasing decisions and mediation
      17, 19

questioning 24, 28, 46
  Rudyard Kipling's six honest serving
      men 35
questions
  closed 46
  open 46
  specific 46

race 76
reflection 24, 58–9, 62, 78
Relate (formerly the Marriage Guidance
      Council) 3
relevance in complaints 23
religion 20, 76
review panel, convening of 9
Rudyard Kipling's six honest serving
      men 35

seeding 36
selfishness, see 'I' factor
setting for meetings 24, 32
   arrangement of chairs in 56
skills, see body language, communication
      skills, note taking
staff
   conciliatory approach of 3
   front line 10, 68–9
   motivation 7
   training 6, 69
stationery, use of by conciliator 16
'story' technique in conciliation 24
'suggestion' 36

'taking sides' 38
'territorial advantage' 31
time 8, 41, 43, 49, 71
   usually taken by mediation 19
timing 70, 74
telephone
   use of in conciliation 24–5
   use of when more than two parties are

      involved 38
training of staff, see staff
trust representative as complained
      against 13

United Nations and mediation 3

values 47, see also attitudes
violence 74
   and health and safety 15
   see also aggression
voice, tone of 48
   see also mouth

Wilson
   Committee 5
   Report ('Being Heard') 5–6
written confirmation by conciliator 37, 77
written word, perception of 37
   see also complaints, written
      acknowledgement of

former Yugoslavia and mediation 3